FAT2FIT

HOW TO MAKE HEALTH AND FITNESS A PART OF YOUR LIFESTYLE

ABHISHEK KUMAR

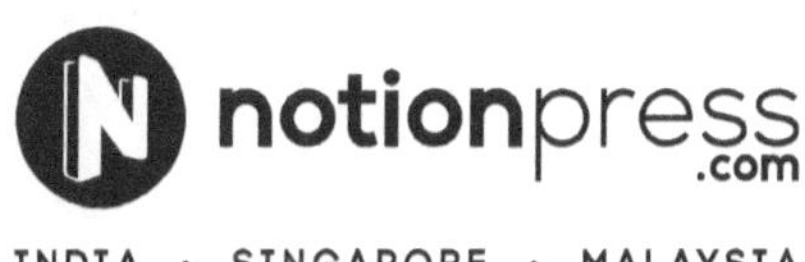

Notion Press Media Pvt Ltd

No. 50, Chettiyar Agaram Main Road,
Vanagaram, Chennai, Tamil Nadu – 600 095

First Published by Notion Press 2021
Copyright © Abhishek Kumar 2021
All Rights Reserved.

ISBN 978-1-63957-405-6

The contents of this book are based on my own thoughts and practices. Any resemblance with anybody regarding this matter is purely coincidental.

Contents

CHAPTER – 1

Daily Hunt Feb Edition

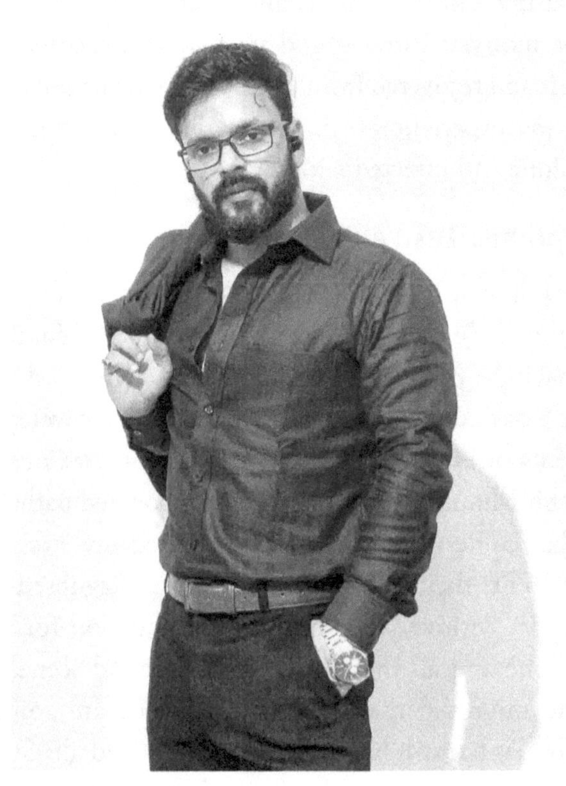

Daily Hunt Article Feb Edition:-

Title: How to stay healthy and Mentally Happy in Quarantine: Gym Freak Abhishek Kumar

Gym Freak Abhishek Kumar from Mumbai recently survived from COVID-19 in the Second Week of April 2021.

Abhishek Kumar says when I was diagnosed with COVID-19. I was very much panicked since I stay alone here at my rented flat in Thane Mumbai. But somehow I have motivated myself and strongly and successfully I faced it and recovered from this. I have taken a call to let's share my experience with society. Especially those who stay alone and infected with COVID.

Symptoms, Test, and Reports

Since I Stay in Mumbai, here are only two seasons rainy or summer. So cold and cough is common in Mumbai. I was having a mild cold I had consulted with my doctors taken 5 day's dose of normal cold and flu. I recovered but suddenly one day's I felt fever I called for a test since 2nd wave hit Mumbai badly. One of the renowned pathology labs has come to my place and collected my swag test. After 36 hrs they send reports that I was diagnosed with Covid-19 Positive. This was a panic situation for me I stay alone and all the news reports and bad scenes run behind my mind that what will happen I am going to die now. What will happen to my family and all? Since I am a Gym freak and health freak. So that self-motivated factor hit me and I have collected all my energy and taken decisions to fight with this and thought will see what will happen.

Don't Panic, face it Think wisely

After test reports, the first thing that came to my mind that I will not go outside in any situation so that I Could not be a corona carrier. I consulted online doctors (lots of App are there). And as per their prescription, I have order medicine using an online App. After that being a responsible citizen I have informed society members where I stay that I have diagnosed covid-19. They appreciate this and did sanitation on my floor outside my house to seal the floor. Then the question was food. I had ordered it through an online app. I was not in the condition to cook, so I have to order Oats, Egg, Tetra pack Milk, Dry fruits, Sprouts, and peanut Butter.

My Full Day Plan

Watchman drops all the material at my doorstep and rings my doorbell. After few minutes I went there and collected my stuff. Then the major challenge was to survive in a 1 bedroom flat for the next 17 days. This hit me again and I was going through lots of things. But again I have collected all my inner energy and started thinking about what can I do. It was a panic situation to stay 17 days in a small area but on another side, it was an opportunity to give yourself time for 17 days. Which is not possible on normal days.

I make a plan after waking up in the morning, went to washroom and finish Brushing my teeth. I did yoga especially Pranayama, Alom Vilom, and Kapalbharti. After that, I used to take bath then do Puja and Dhayan. Doing Puja and Dhayan gives inner peace and positive vibes. You can be of any religion but putting some time for prayers it gives us lots of energy. After Dhayan I do my breakfast.

I have to take Sprouts and dry fruits on daily coz it's contain full of energy diet then medicine. After that I take my phone and search for my contact details in thousands of numbers was saved on my phone you won't believe I connected to lots of my friends during my school time and college time. I have connected to lots of my family members whom I haven't connected.

Since long, after doing all family and friends sessions. I prepared lunch for myself. It was milk mix with water and oats. This was my lunch and after Lunch, I post my old workout video on my social media account. Which I use to do during the lockdown last year. I got a good response I have seen people are needed that they need to know to do workout at home they asked for a diet plan also. Believe me, I helped many people without charging a single penny. Daily I had started posting one video doing the workout at home and helping others to do the same. Out of which few became best friends of mine. After that, I take 3-4 white eggs in evening snacks.

Family

After all my friends and Social media stuff I start talking to my family members my parents my sisters and in-laws in the evening it helps me to understand them and at the same time, it gives me the courage to face covid-19 strongly. They were very concern and panic for me. But my daily phone makes them relax that I am fine. Family play a key role in our life so you should always communicate with family on daily basis, they deserve our time. Covid-19 has taught us that life is unpredictable so enjoy its every moment. After conversations with family and parents, I prepare dinner for myself a brown bread with peanut butter and Turmeric milk.

I am completed my quarantine days and I am absolutely fine

Summary

So I will suggest everyone, don't be panic behave wisely.

*Don't see anything negative, negative always impacts your mind badly. So stop watching the news the entire day for sake of information. Listen music it will help you to be happy, sleep early and wake up early. Believe me that, Time will not be going to come back again so enjoy each and every moment of your life. Don't take lightly to these viruses criticizing our system is always easy But we should responsible for ourselves and our family first. No one will come to save us this is our responsibility to save ourselves and our family and friends. Same time don't misbehave with covid-19 patient treat them well and motivate them morally at least.

*Keep social distance.

*Wash your hand regularly and use a mask and sanitizer.

* In situations of staying home do some Dhayan and yoga, it will help your mind to be happy.

* Do daily what you love more. I was doing a home workout with No equipment or very minimum equipment.

Let's pray we will recover from this situation of covid-19 soon. And please takes care of yourself and your dearest and nearest one. Don't take it lightly but same time don't be panic.

CHAPTER – 2

Influencive Article can Search Abhishek Kumar Fitness at Google

Influencive article May 2021

One better thing happened that I got an inspiration and Idea to launch my fitness platform to help the needy but at a minimal cost. And this inspired me to write about my transformation journey and many others who did their transformation.

Idea Behind writing this book and launching fitness platform nagafitness.com for the needy came from: -

Before covid-19 (Nov 2019) my cholesterol level was 264 and my weight was approximately 90 kg. It was an alarming situation for me. I went to a very good MD practitioner near me and discuss my health report. He suggested not to have cholesterol medicine or else have to take it for lifetimes. He suggested doing a workout and have a healthy diet and proper rest. Or else I could have heart disease soon. It was an alarming situation for me

I have started doing workouts taking a Proper diet and proper sleep in the next 4months I lose around 20kg.

I did lots of research on diet and workout I never followed or purchase any diet plan I customized my own and got results.

In March 2020. We all have seen the first lockdown and everything was closed I have worked hard for my weight loss and never was in the mood to waste all those things by sitting at home. I have discussed with my younger sister and we both started doing homework out together she lost around 16 kg in 3 months. And I succeeded to maintain my weight.

Now I am helping others to achieve their goal online through phone calls, video calls, and also live workout sessions, weight loss is very easy when you are dedicated to it and it will not easy when you are lazy. Lots of Peoples are enjoying their transformation.

Homework Out:-

Homework out is mainly for general fitness and basic bodybuilding. And this is very much required for old age people, busy and working professionals and housewife who is not able to go the gym. But in current situations when we are saying to stay home and be safe, in this situation home workout is necessary for everyone. You can check any interview of doctors they are recommending to Do Daily workouts in these pandemic times.

Workout helps you to increase immunity in your body, digestion and proper respiration and blood circulation workout. It will help you to maintain proper oxygen levels in your body.

Now the people are facing the challenges that "how to do a workout "And "When to do workout see everyone has different lifestyles and Different professions. Some work out do in the morning, some in the afternoon and some in the evening or night so there can't be a perfect schedule time for the workout. Everyone should do it in a fixed time as per their convenience. As per their working and different lifestyle. But try to fix the same time to achieve the best results.

Now the question is How and which Workout???

See everyone have different body structure and different Problem so each and every one can customize their workout plan, by discussing with their trainer. For example, we can do push-ups, skipping jumping squats lunges crunches without any equipment. And with the support of extension rope so we can perform the entire workout. I am not against of gym in this pandemic situation and the people who don't have time basically the female of our family or the older Family members can't go outside or not willing to go outside for workout they can perform at home with proper guidance and support.

Homework Out Motivation:-

Motivation plays a crucial role in any development, we know how the world is accepting motivational speakers nowadays for development. Some people are self-motivated some need motivation. So home workout.

Motivation is a much-needed thing for better results always try to contact those who have done all those things and gone through all those things. You need to care for yourself, you have to love yourself. Give some time to yourself for better grooming in all aspects.

Diet:-

Diet is very much important in any transformation. We can spend our 1hrs only one hours time for workout on Daily basis but main body transformation depends on our kitchen what we eat how much we eat etc. Now people will ask what to eat and how much see everyone have different taste and they want to eat as per their taste and like some are pure veg some like nonveg some have Jain food in taste. So believe me you can customize your diet with the proper dietitian. It will help you to enjoy your transformation. And as per body types and requirements also you can customize your diet plan.

Some needs to lose same line needs to weight gain so diet will be varied to the person to person so people should work and customize their diet plan with the help of their dietitian.

Transformation:-

Here I would like to say that body transformation is not about losing weight only weight gain is also coming under body transformation and believe me losing weight is tough but gaining weight is tougher.

Read and see the body transformation journey of people it will motivate you and challenge you to achieve your best. Once you will come in contact with people who transformed them you will see the difference in their physical appearance, in their body language their confidence level, and their testosterone levels. And this will motivate to do workout and transform yourself.

Family workout:-

Pandemic has taught us that life is unpredictable and you are most loved and cared for by your family members only. So being a responsible Family member we should encourage or motivate our family members to do the workout. It will create a good and positive environment in the home it will support and motivate other family members to do workouts and other hand it increases love affection bonding and caring in the family. Especially ladies members of our family who are the backbone of the family including mother grandmother sister-wife daughters

They are not made to just do household work they also deserve healthy Life.

Take care of your family members especially Female members so that they Take care of us in the best and better manners.

CHAPTER – 3

Anupama Transformation

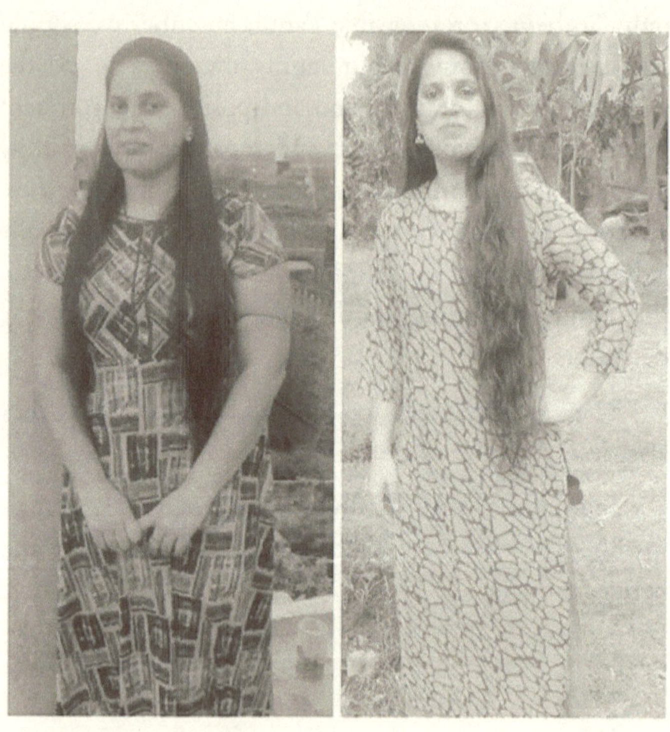

Transformations Stories:-

Anupama Transformation A brain behind NAGA Fitness.Com

It is not about being perfect. It's about effort. When you implement that effort into your life, every single day, that's where transformation happens, says Anupama Kumari whose transformation story is truly an inspirational one. Read her story and derive inspiration for your fitness journey.

Anupama Kumari is a mathematician teacher by Profession. She was suffering from overweight she had put on so much weight and started getting troubled with problem of thyroid. That made her panic. But one day she decided to join the gym and started following a healthy diet. So she would say that she herself and her body inspired her to get fit and healthy.

Anupama exercise 1years ago with a goal to be fit. With a dedicated diet and hard training, she was able to achieve 16kg weight lose within 45 days. Since then, she decided to focus upon to help others who wants to lose weight.

There were so many challenges before she decided to step on stage because she comes from a very small town that is Dhanbad Jharkhand. There she wasn't allowed to wear jeans and basic t-shirts. But yes she was a kid who always wanted to do something different from other kids. Since childhood she was a sporty person and loved to play all outdoor activities. But when she got rejection in her marriage, then her parents supported her for workout and body weight transformation. Anupama Kumari successfully made her family proud of her achievements. She faced one more challenge during her body weight transformation which was the biggest challenge her hypo thyroid. She taken proper diet and proper workout to defeat all the obstacle. And this transformation motivate her to launch a fitness platform for needy.

She writes in her website of NAGA Fitness.Com;-

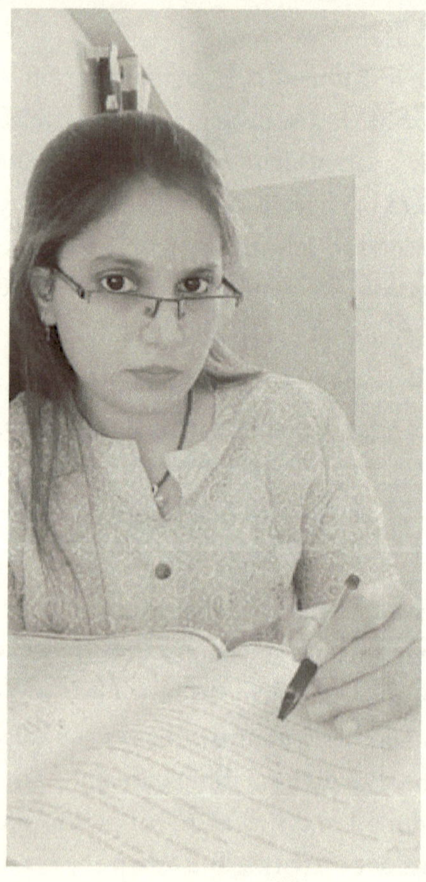

I am Anupama a mathematician, and a teacher by profession. Specialty in Child development phycology. I have diversified my career in Health and fitness and launch this platform to help others.

Many people ask me what was idea and motivation behind to launch this platform??

See I am from a middle class traditional background family. A family who was always involve in social welfare of needy always.

I have completed my schooling staying with my parents. Actually in middle class family parents behave like teacher they try to make their daughter a super woman so that after marriage she can perform her best role towards her in-law's husband and their family.

So after my school and collage I was working with my mother and was helping her in kitchen and other household work. And after that I was busy in my studies and assignment. Was hardly giving time to my health, my weight was increasing day by day. I have not think on that actually in middle class family hardly people think of health, health is least priority and the last priority in their monthly budget. In fact, the thought of health is for richer or upper middle class people, is coming from middle class people only.

After doing my Bachelor in Education and post-graduation in mathematics, my parents start searching groom for me who can take care of myself lifelong. Highly focused and dreamed area of a parents is to marry their daughter, during these process I got lots of rejection due to my weight.

This was the first time when I have realised I am fat but for others parents are like no she is healthy no fat. But fact was that I was facing rejection at that time.

This was the time my elder brother was working for his transformation and was posting us about his journey and was motivating us to do the same. I got idea and requested her to help me out, I have joint him and started working towards my transformation. I have joined him but after doing workout and diet in 20 days I was not able to lose single kg. This was again frustrating for me but my mentor and teacher my brother told my no worries transformation will happen. After that we came to know that I was suffering from Hypo thyroid, and question was now I will do? It was my brother who told me will do keep patience, believe me I haven't taken online diet plan, it was brother deep knowledge of diet and workout that helps to reduce my weight. So after I tested for hypo thyroid brother change my diet plan and we started again for the transformation. After next in two months I have loose around 16kg. I was so happy my family friends all appreciated this.

I was thinking due to my brother I have done my transformation, what about others once you stared going gym people will ask to take protein powder without knowing your health condition, without knowing your budget.

From there I got idea and motivation to launch a fitness platform from where I can motivate and helps other to do the same. I have launched NAGA fitness.com for the needy people.

Regards Anupma.

Here she shares her basic workout regime:

I work out 6 days a week. Every day I target different part of the body with 1/2 hour cardio daily like:

- Glutes

- Shoulders

- Back

- Glutes

- Shoulders

- Triceps and biceps

Here she shares her basic diet:

- 5 meals in a day and each meal includes portion of protein, carbohydrates, veggies and fats.

- Supplements like fish oil and multivitamins.

With regards to time management to stay fit Anupama says, "Being a middle class daughter it's difficult to manage all the things sometimes, but as we say, where there is a will, there is a way. But I love my family and I have passion at the same time. I learned the skills to manage my time and I always make sure I should have all meals on time. Sometimes I keep my diet flexible especially when I'm traveling but I always focus on eating healthy. I also believe in good spiritual health so I meditate daily to keep my mind stable, healthy and positive."

In her message to the people who want to transform, Anupama Says," transformation isn't sweet and bright, it's dark and murky, painful pushing. It's not about being perfect. It's about effort. And when you implement that effort into your life, every single day, that's where transformation happens. That's how change occurs. Keep going and remember why you started."

CHAPTER – 4

Anuradha Transformation

She was Body Shamed Yet Transformed: Anuradha Fitness Journey

There are many people who wish to live to the fullest and not fall into the 'discipline' trap. The carefree attitude, however, weighs heavy on them over the period of time. But Anuradha realized the need to change just in time and pledged a fit lifestyle for the rest of her life!

I am Anuradha Singh a 30-year-old from Durgapur west Bangal. I am currently preparing for a general competition. And a mother of a kid.

I started gaining weight in my graduation tremendously due to unhealthy eating habits and no physical exercises. I used to eat a lot of junk food. Then, in my graduation days, parties, eating outside and all was a part of my lifestyle. As a result, I gained lot of weight in that time period.

I used to get negative comments on my body type, made fun about every single thing and that was the most depressing part. Believe me body shaming can break anyone's confidence. I was depressed in those years and I used to cry a lot, questioned myself why I am this way. I used to binge eat after starving whole day in order to lose weight.

My transformation journey did not happen overnight, no one can transform the body without the correct mind set. In Jan 2020, I decided to work on myself honestly. But prior to that, I tried lots of crash diets and all but nothing worked. So I started all over again with small steps with the help of NAGA Fitness. com. My only goal at that time was to lose weight. There were many hurdles, in initial weeks I used to get frustrated easily because I was working very hard but couldn't see any results, so with patience and consistency my hard work paid off, I saw myself transforming not only by body but by my mind set, my strength and everything got build up.

In initial days, I had no knowledge about anything. In the whole phase, So I started with running and cardio. After developing enough strength, later on, I added weight training.

Nutrition plays the most important role, so my diet basically includes veggies, lentils, salad, oatmeal, whole food soy, protein shakes, and fruit salad. I cheat once in a while. My workout schedule is 6 days of weight training (2 muscle groups), like legs with shoulder, chest with triceps, back with biceps and ½ hour of running, sprints and then some core exercises. I go for outdoor running on off days. I am not saying it is going to be easy, but it is always worth it.

Thanks to Naga Fitness.Com.

CHAPTER – 5

Abhishek Kumar
Transformation

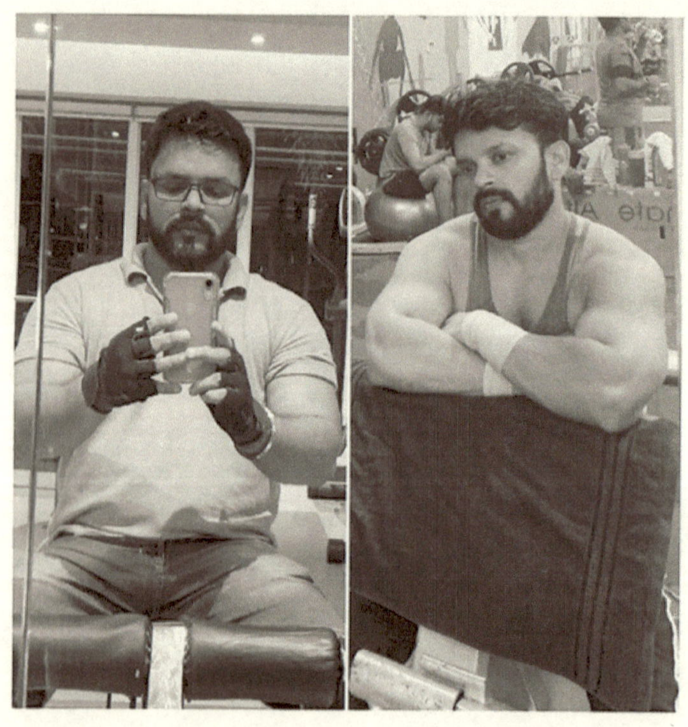

Abhishek Kumar Transformation Journey

My cholesterol level was 264, and my weight was approximately 90 kg. It was an alarming situation for me. I went to a very good MD practitioner near me and discuss my health report. He suggested not to have cholesterol medicine or else have to take it for lifetimes. He suggested doing a workout and have a healthy diet and proper rest. Or else I could have heart disease soon. It was an alarming situation for me I have started doing workouts taking a Proper diet and proper sleep in the next 4months I lose around 20kg.

I did lots of research on diet and workout I never followed or purchase any diet plan I customized my own and got results.

In March 2020. We all have seen the first lockdown and everything was closed I have worked hard for my weight loss and never was in the mood to waste all those things by sitting at home. I have discussed with my younger sister and we both started doing homework out together she lost around 16 kg in 3 months. And I succeeded to maintain my weight.

Now I am helping others to achieve their goal online through phone calls, video calls, and also live workout sessions, weight loss is very easy when you are dedicated to it and it will not easy when you are lazy. Lots of Peoples are enjoying their transformation. Remaining already mention in my Article with Influencive in May. You can refer chapter 2.

CHAPTER – 6

Role of Diet in Transformation

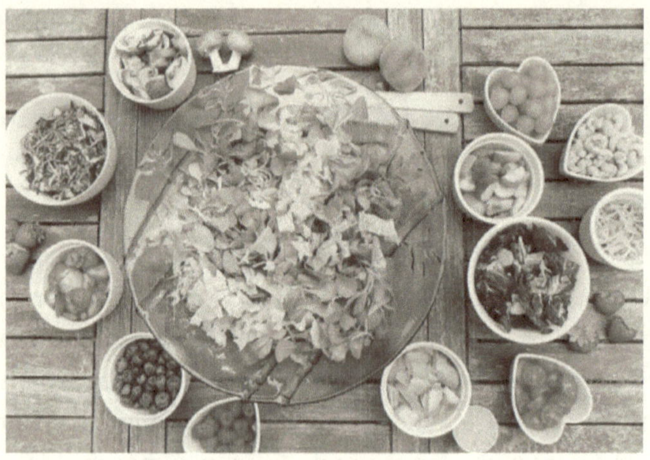

Diet:-

Diet plays an important role in body weight transformation, experts say it plays a Seventy percent role in any body transformation. People who know me always say that you can't lose weight I was foody. But when I have decided to transform myself I have taken care of my diet. Diet is not eating less it is always eating right. Calories deficit food is much necessary when we are in plan to lose weight. I have started cutting my carbs increase my protein and fibre intake with natural resources. Boiled egg, boiled chicken, sprouts these food was major sources of protein for me. And for good fats I used to cooked food in olive oil, then for fibre, I was depended on cabbage, Guava, and some often I used to have Papaya also. I was taking food every 2-3 hours, for sure.

My interest in nutrition began during my transformation. I haven't purchase or taken any diet plan from anyone. I have make a diet plan for myself after doing lots of research and as per my choice. I remember before I started my transformation, I was doing party eating anything, I was 90kg at that point of time, My coaches say that my body is natural I haven't taken any supplements. I have transformed myself from 90 kg to 68 kg. In 4 months, discipline dedication, and guide of my coach. I used no supplements, protein shakes and proper food, and the plan I followed was far from restrictive, The exercise regimen I stuck to was something I enjoyed and followed in a controlled manner. There was no over-exercising. There was no looking for shorts cuts, no complaint about how tough it was or blaming it on hormones, motherhood, being a working and busy professionals, etc. I have focused to do or have to do. After doing lots of research on Indian food spices, herbs, beverages, nuts, and seeds that could prevent and maybe even cure the deadliest of diseases, help burn fats, improve energy levels, detoxify the liver, colon, and blood, and boost immunity? It was then that I realized how blessed we are. we live in a country where we had access to some of the most nutritious food in the world most of the world now has access to Indian food, thanks to advanced technology and advanced logistics. We have everything in our own country, and if used in the right way it can prevent and cure diseases and possibly, alter the country's health statistics. Normally we are completely convinced that the Mediterranean, diet with its staples of fruits, vegetables, whole grains legumes, and nuts indigenous to the region, was the healthiest in the world. It is healthy; there is no doubt about that, but when I decide to break it down in detail and compare it with the Indian diet, we began to believe and are now completely convinced, that the Indian diet is as healthy, or might we say even healthiest than the Mediterranean diet. Every country or region will have a diet that is local and healthy for the people that live there. The Mediterranean diet will perhaps be healthy for people living in the Mediterranean region, as the Chinese diet, would be healthy, for those in China. There is a lot of extremely healthy food that is common to almost all cuisines globally.

Plant-Based Foods:-

A recent survey suggests that we are starting to shun meaty roasts and bangers in favour of healthier. Plant-Based swaps. More and more people are eating more vegetables, fruits. Soya and nut products than a few years ago. Mostly, it is younger consumers aged between 18 and 30. Who is turning to alternative, more sustainable ways of eating?

Enjoying the benefits of more plant-based choices doesn't mean becoming Vegan or vegetarian. It's about reshaping what's on your plate and making simple swaps, while still treating yourself to favourite meat or dairy products when your fancy them- instead of eating them from habit. Even cutting down on half, your intake of meat and dairy will make a considerable impact on your health and environment. For example, it takes over 2400 gallons, of water to produce one pound of meat. 2000 gallons of water to produce one gallon of milk, but an average of 25 gallons of water to produce one pound of plant-based food.

The latest international nutrition guidelines also aim to increase people's intake of seafood and fat-free and low-fat milk and milk products and consume only moderate amounts of lean meat, poultry, and eggs.

An herb Garden:-

Now is the perfect time to plant an herb garden in your home. Everyone is seated in lockdown searching for what to do in lockdown. This is a better idea to help the environment and help yourself. I have learned planting and gardening with my grandfather at my native, there I was a huge space for gardening. This is an ideal time to plan your plantings and installing a selection of herbs can transform your meals, save money, and have medicinal benefits. Transform a small patch of land near your kitchen door (for ease of access when cooking) or go to town with a larger, impressive traditional herb garden in the form of a medieval knot. And if you don't have a garden, you can still grow herbs in window boxes, patio pots, or tubs by your front door. They are easy to cultivate and look attractive, too.

Lavender:-

Acts as soothing. Calming sedatives to relax the mind. Promote sleep and ward off headaches.

German Chamomile: -

Flowers and leaves are used to make a medicinal tea that can improve indigestion, wind and promote a good night's sleep. Soak cotton pads in cooled chamomile tea to bathe tired, strained eyes.

Lemon Balm:-

Was a popular remedy for stress in medieval times, when scholars facing exams chewed its leaves, also helps indigestion, flatulence, and anxiety.

Sage:-

Is it one of the most versatile medicinal herbs? As well as making sage and onion stuffing. You can rub fresh sage leaves onto insect stings and bites, or make an infusion to gargle away a sore throat or ease menopausal hot flushes. Freezing sage leaves retains their medicinal benefits better than drying.

Mint:-

Is one of the most popular garden herbs, and is often grown in pots to curtail its invasive nature. Its leaves contain essentials oils with antiseptic and painkilling properties, and it makes the most wonderful, herbal tisane. Perfect for improving digestion-just add 1- Tablespoon mint leaves to a cup of boiling water and infuse for 20 minutes before drinking.

Benefits of growing your herbs:-

1. Fresh flavours are always available to liven salads, pasta, pizzas, and meats in summer and dried or frozen herbs can be used throughout winter.

2. Save money all year round- even small bags of herb are expensive to buy fresh out of season.

3. Improve the curb appeal of your home-a well-tended kitchen herb patch looks attractive (especially if you are looking to sell your home).

4. Homemade gifts are always available lavender sachets, fresh poise, or dried bouquet grain mixes.

5. Relieve the stresses and strains of daily life-tending your home-grown herbs and inhaling their wonderful scent will both relax and revitalize you at the end of a long working day.

CHAPTER – 7

Timing of Workout

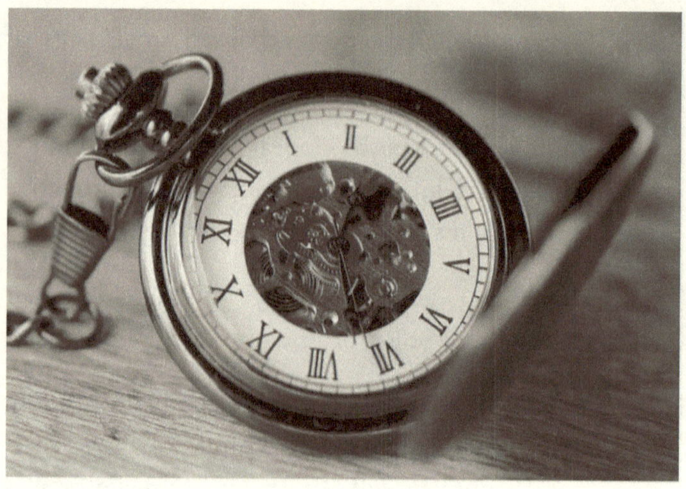

When we should do the workout:-

See doing the workout is most important than its timing, but most people are day routine I mean they work in the morning to evening shift. So if you have time and you are morning evening shift guys please wake up early. We all grow up by listening to that poem early to bed, early to rise makes a man healthy wealthy, and wise. Most successful people support the philosophy of waking up early and doing the workout. Wake up early have some hot water wear sports clothes take your phone and headphone. Listen to your favourite songs music speech whatever you like, can you imagine every morning its exciting isn't it.

Waking up early gives you extra time to work on yourself. It allows you to give time to yourself and do something for your betterment.

Early to bed and early to rise makes one healthy, wealthy and wise. This saying taught in primary school is one of the most important learnings, relevant throughout our life. According to research, enough sleep and waking up early helps the body and mind get enough relaxation. It is also very important for maintaining the overall health of the body. We bring a few benefits of waking up early.

Peace and solace: According to the research, when you wake up early before the rest of the world wakes up you have peaceful moments for yourself. There is no heavy honking from the traffic or neighbours speaking loudly. Early mornings are a great relaxation time. You can step out of the house to get some fresh air, prepare yourself. According to science the silent moments are highly beneficial for the brain and body; they help in increasing the oxygen levels in the brain, reduce blood pressure, lessen migraines, and boost mental health.

Enough time for breakfast: Usually when people tend to wake up late, they grab a portion of cereal with lots of sugar, or drink some beverage and rush to work. Breakfast is considered the most important meal of the day considering the huge health benefits it offers like improves metabolism to burn calories, provides sufficient energy for the day, lowers bad cholesterol, reduces the risk of diabetes and heart diseases, limits the chance of becoming overweight and boosts mood and positive thinking.

Better brain function: According to the research, people who wake up early have better brain function, superior critical thinking, and problem-solving skills. Such people also tend to be more humorous with a lot of positive energy and likely to deeply engage themselves with. Sleeping early and waking up early improves concentration and memory power too. This means people will tend to perform better at work and the children in their studies.

Waking up early provides more energy: People who have fewer hours of sleep experience low levels of energy and negativity. They also experience mood swings and temper tantrums. Furthermore, they overindulge in sweet eating to ease their moods. This is not good for health. By gathering a good night's sleep and waking up early one can benefit from it since the body provides more energy. It also helps in the proper functioning of the body that includes increased supply in blood muscles, tissue repairs, bone repair, lowered blood pressure, and relaxation of the body.

Waking early makes you look more attractive: Waking up early can help you improve your appearance. Sleeping and waking late can make you feel and look more tired. Also, less sleep brings puffiness and dark circles around the eyes. According to the research, people who sleep and wake up early look fresh and beautiful. People, who are planning to lose weight, also should wake up early and have breakfast at the right time.

Morning Exercise: Morning is considered to be the best time for workouts and exercises. Most of us have tightly scheduled mornings and there is no time to hit the gym, walk or practice fitness schedules. Waking up early gives you enough time to exercise in the mornings and follow your fitness regime. There's nothing like a great workout to boost your day and feel rejuvenated.

Keeps lifestyle diseases at bay: According to medical experts, lifestyle-related diseases such as obesity, thyroid, and polycystic ovarian syndrome are caused due to stress, lack of exercise, and poor diet. Getting proper sleep can relax the body and also help in the normal production of hormones. Proper sleep cycles are required in the overall smooth functioning of all the organs of the body.

Bigger scores: According to research conducted by Texas University students who were early risers scored better grades than those who were late to rise. Students are engaged with their studies and assignments all day and exhausted at the end of the day, sleeping and waking up early gives their body and mind gets adequate rest, and a fresh mind will help them study well and achieve high grades.

Easier commutes: A little delay can upset morning commutes and make traffic-intensive. Especially in metropolitan cities. Waking up early and leaving to work early will certainly ease the delays. Taking time on the way to work lowers the stress, and allows relaxing and thinking about work, and the rest of the day's schedule.

More family time: Usually when things do not go according to the schedules, towards the latter end of the day, we get preoccupied with the shortcomings. However, when you wake up early and things go according to plan, there is a greater level of satisfaction that comes at the end of the day. Despite being tired from the day's work you can unwind in the company of those you love in a relaxed ambiance.

CHAPTER – 8

Perspiration
(Heavy Sweating)

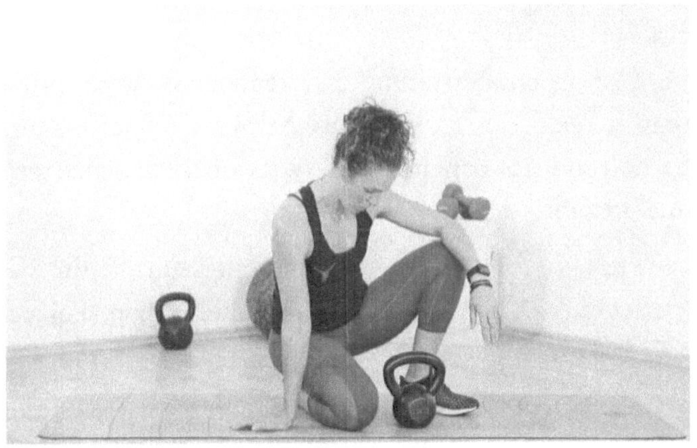

Perspiration myth vs reality:-

Excess sweating is a common and embarrassing problem. In many cases it is a normal and temporary response to exercise, vigorous dancing, being hot, or emotionally stressed. For one in hundred people, however, excess sweating leads to constant wet patches, embarrassment, loss of confidence, and a fear of the body, odour. The good news is that the problem can usually be overcome with a little Know-How.

How to reduce sweating

Avoid man-made fibres such as nylon, instead wear natural fabrics such as cotton which let sweat evaporate more easily.

Use an absorbent powder on your feet and in body creases to soak up any excess sweat. If you are prone to fungal skin infections, such as Athlete's foot, use an antifungal powder and dust it inside your shoes and socks as well.

Use an antiperspirant that reduces sweating rather than a deodorant, which just helps to reduce odours. Some products contain both types of ingredients for a dual benefit.

Freshen up underarms and going during the day if necessary- Carry a wash kit (flannels, Soap, Powder, towel) with you.

Carry a change of clothes if necessary for instant freshness during the day.

Powerful antiperspirants containing aluminium chloride hex hydrate, are available from pharmacies to control sweating in problem areas. Follow instructions, but generally, they are applied to clean, dry skin at night- when sweat glands are inactive and washed off the next morning. The solution can be used on any area prone to excessive sweating that comes under control, applications can be reduced in frequency to once or twice a week.

Most people find that the above tips together with a thorough wash, shower, or bath at least once a day, and after vigorous exercise keep sweating under control. If you continue to have problems with excessive sweating. In some cases, for example, it may be a sign of an overactive thyroid gland or a hidden infection. Overactive sweat glands can be treated medically with injections of botulinum toxin or if necessary, surgery to cut the nerves supplying sweat glands in problem areas.

Tamarind seeds and their flowers are also known to make a good home remedy against excessive perspiration. Take a few tamarind seeds along with a tamarind flower, soak in water and grind them together to form a paste. Apply it to the places most affected. It also deals with body odour effectively.

Eating right also helps you manage excessive sweating. Food high in zinc helps reduce the formation of sweet and sweaty odour. Such foods include whole grains, nuts, and legumes. Try and avoid foods like fish and garlic, which make your sweating smell really bad.

Use a deodorant that is alum-based because alum controls sweating and reduce offensive body odour. You could also rub an easily available alum crystal. However, make sure you smoothen the edges before using them on your skin.

CHAPTER – 9

No Pain No Gain

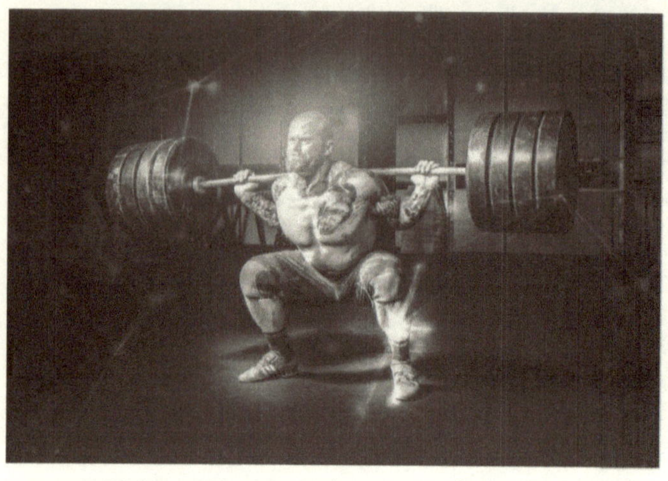

No Pain no grain is universal truth. You can correlate with any context of your life. It's not just a statement it is a truth especially when it's come to fitness context. No, why it's painful when we do the workout. Muscular soreness associated with exercise usually comes in two waves. First is occurs pain or burn, you feel while you are working out. And for short time afterward. Then within twenty-four hours of your exercise session, you may experience delayed onset muscle, soreness, and stiffness that's the pain you feel when getting out of bed the morning after a tough workout. Interestingly, no single physical mechanism is universally accepted as the cause of muscle soreness. Several theories have been suggested over the last hundreds of years. But the most popular idea, that it's due to a build-up. Of lactic acid now seems less likely in the light of recent studies. The most likely causes of acute muscle soreness are now thought to include muscle fatigue, and tissue swelling from blood fluids passing into muscle tissues. However most of the pain you experience after exercise-especially the delayed onset muscle soreness- is thought to results from micro trauma or tiny tears in muscle fibres.

Don't let the thought of muscle tears put you off, exercise, however, your body adapts to this damage by not only repairing the tears but by building additional tissue in an attempt, to prevent it from happening again. Many weightlifters view micro trauma as a positive part of their exercise plans, as it plays a part in actively promoting muscle growth.

Now when you exercise vigorously and particularly if it's a new exercise that works different muscles a degree of muscle soreness is inevitable. However, there are steps you can take to keep pain to a minimum and to speed your recovery afterward.

Get enough rest, while you sleep your body repairs those minuscule tears that are causing pain, Aim for a good seven to eight hours of sleep in the days following a strenuous workout session.

Remain well-hydrated drinking plenty of water helps to flush out toxins and your muscles heal more easily, Poor hydration on the other hand may exacerbate the soreness. And also contributes to painful muscles cramp.

Perform light exercise. Walking a light jog or swimming may seem counterintuitive, but it promotes the circulation of oxygen-rich blood, to your muscle fibres, helping to relieve pain and to shorten the recovery time for sore muscles, this is sometimes, known as active recovery, and is highly recommended as a natural and positive way to reduce pain.

Finally, if the pain is severe, you may want to use non-steroidal anti-inflammatory drugs such as aspirin or a topical pain gel or cream designed for muscle pain, however, it's important to remember that these only relieve pain, and are not designed to speed recovery. Use of such products should be the exception don't rely on them to ease exercise pain on a frequent or recurring basis.

CHAPTER – 10

Health and Lifestyle

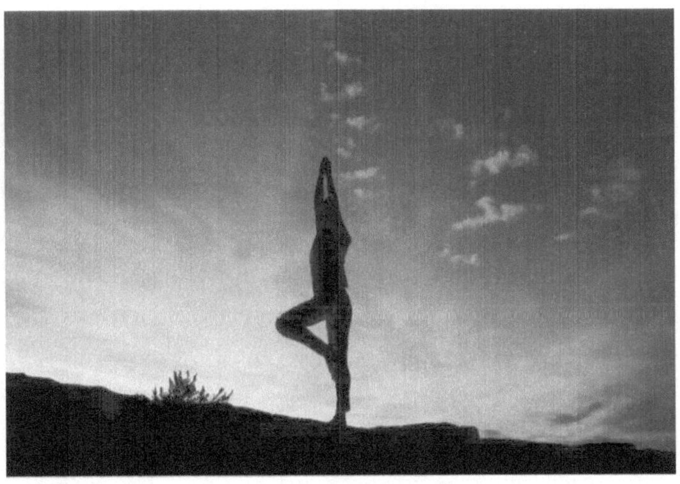

Lifestyle and workout Habits:-

There is plenty of evidence of habits and certain lifestyle factors. Can significantly affect how sore you feel after exercise. Unsurprisingly overall fitness plays a big part- if you only exercise infrequently. You are more likely to experience muscular soreness than if you are fit and work out regularly. Good dietary habits also help. Try to maintain healthy nutrition, nutritional balance, paying particular attention to protein intake and mineral-like potassium, which the body uses to build and maintain healthy muscles. Antioxidants found in fruit and veg are also. Important to reduce inflammation and damage. If you are not eating a healthy diet, you will find that the muscle soreness takes longer to heal.

Workout and Brain health:-

Recent studies often talk about mental health and physical health, but it is necessary to look for both of them together. Generally, mental health can be defined as how people feel, think and act when faced with life's problems. In addition, a mental disease causes feelings of unhappiness, loss of hope, sleeping problems, changes in eating habits, loss of interest in natural activities, and pains that have no physical description. Occasionally, mental and physical illnesses appear similar in many symptoms, such as a decrease in food cravings and energy levels. Therefore, this essay aims to argue specific situations could affect both mental and physical health. This essay will consider depression, exercise, humour, and environment respectively. Depression is one of the most popular mental diseases in the world. It is a feeling of sadness and low self-esteem, which is experienced by someone over a long period; also, it can change physical health, behaviour, and appearance. Roughly, 450 million people are afflicted by depression worldwide as well it attacks one out of every five people throughout their lifetime in some countries (World Health Organization, 2001). In addition, mood can be influenced by lifestyle, past experiences, and genetic factors (BBC website cited in Woodward, 2014). Generally, depression can be treated with antidepressants, psychological therapies, or a mixture of both. Nevertheless, antidepressants may have opposing side effects and adherence can be poor (Mead, et al., 2009). One of the secrets of mental stability is avoiding negative opinions, which is being able to notice when you are 'choosing' or 'allowing yourself to think positively rather than negatively (BBC website cited in Woodward, 2014). Besides, they say that the persons who continually appear to be in a good mood have higher levels of hormone endorphins, neurotransmitters dopamine, and serotonin. These are secreted by the brain and make people feel good when they are enjoying themselves or when something nice occurs.

Exercise and physical activity are linked to a higher quality of life and health. Numerous scientists researched on this subject and all of them found out a significant correlation between physical activity and mental health, but they have differed in what kind, when, how, and how many exercises are needed. Experts say that exercise improves mood and decreases symptoms of anxiety and depression. They show that people diagnosed with depression undergoing an aerobic exercise intervention exhibited great improvements in depression compared to people who received only psychotropic treatment. In addition, another study suggests that practicing at least 60-150 minutes per week of intermediate to energetic physical activity, inhibits depression and boosts good mental health. Conversely, one report states that more than a hundred scientific studies dealing with exercise and mental health, and not all of these studies show statistically important benefits with exercise training indicate that the link between exercise and higher levels of life was no causal, and mediated by genetic factors that affect both exercise behaviour and well-being. They go on to say that physical activity and positive happiness, which appear to be independent risk factors for health. For these reasons, regular exercise is connected with better mental health, although there is a lack of consensus about the optimal volume and nature of the activity to accomplish these benefits.

Many pieces of research show that a good sense of humour works as a good 'immunity medicine', raising resistance to disease. According to these researches, the capability to see the funny aspect of things enhances both physical and mental well-being. Experts says that, "the best clinicians understand that there is an intrinsic physiological intervention brought about by positive emotions such as mirthful laughter, optimism, and hope. Lifestyle choices have a significant impact on health and disease and these are choices which the patient exercises control relative to prevention and treatment. They approve that laughter and humour may not work out life's troubles, however, it does set people in a better place to tackle them. These examples show that laughter helps to relax the body by decreasing blood pressure and tension in the muscles.

The environment has large effects on the mental and physical health of humans. It is more challenging to be physically active while living in an insecure or unhealthy region. researches states that housing insecurity may be especially stressful and bring on poorer mental and physical health. Research shows that mental disease can affect social and cognitive function and reduce energy levels, which can negatively affect the adoption of healthy behaviours. People may lack the motivation to look after their health; moreover, they may take unhealthy eating and sleeping habits, smoke or abuse substances, as an effect or reaction to their symptoms, contributing to worse health effects. One such study demonstrates that people living in low-income families are more likely to hurt mental health problems than their wealthier peers. For these reasons, people living with higher penury, jobless, lack of stable housing, and social isolation, are higher susceptible to mental and physical illnesses.

To summarise, mental and physical health are inextricably linked. A large number of studies have encouraged that practicing at a minimal level of at least 60 minutes/week of any physical activity, and take enough humour time in a nice place that will help to have a healthy body and mind. Although more accurate studies are required, to prove what kind and how physical activity demand for each specific illness.

How to Create Mind Set of Workout

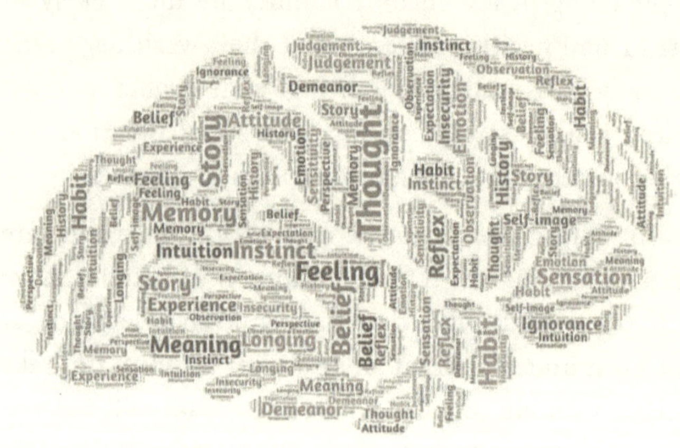

Train Your Mind for the workout:-

If your fitness routine has been less than consistent over the past few months, you're likely not alone. Summer is a unique season: longer days often consist of making after-work plans with friends, taking family vacations, and spending weekends at outdoor barbecues or the beach — not hours logged inside a gym.

And while the warm weather does provide ample opportunity to be active outdoors, a more erratic schedule can make it difficult to schedule it inconsistently. Now that fall is here and work and family obligations tend to fall back in line, we can make fitness a more consistent part of our routine again.

But after a few lax months, this is easier said than done. Anyone who has tried to lose weight, tone up, or even just simply recommit to exercise knows that the battle is often more mental than physical. So I tapped some of my experience of my personal training, for some advice on how it helps my clients to overcome from their mental hurdle. Here are some of their best mental hacks to get your mind in the game — and your body back in the shape.

Start with mini workouts

Your normal plan of attack is likely to hit the ground running, scheduling hour-long workout sessions a few days a week. But experts say to start small. We're talking 5-minute workout small.

"I tell my weight-loss clients who are not used to working out that they need to start with a mini-workout," It is an immediate way to combat any excuse you may have on why you can't exercise — after all, who doesn't have five minutes to spare? "Some people say, 'I don't have 30 minutes to work out; I can't even get to the gym; where do I start?' Start with a mini workout — literally 5 minutes,"

It could crunch while you're watching TV, squats while you fold the laundry, or a walk around the block. "It sounds gimmicky but these are the types of movements that you want to start doing so you get that muscle memory," "In your mind, you're seeing the workout as just five minutes and who knows? You may be inspired to go for five more minutes and that will build and build."

This mental hack is twofold. First, it's easier to convince yourself to do something for five minutes rather than 30, especially if you've been off your workout grind for a while. Beyond that, you are slowly starting to condition your mind to put health front and centre and getting your body used to moving, which will help build motivation over time.

CHAPTER – 12

6 Mental Tricks that Help Make Exercise a Habit

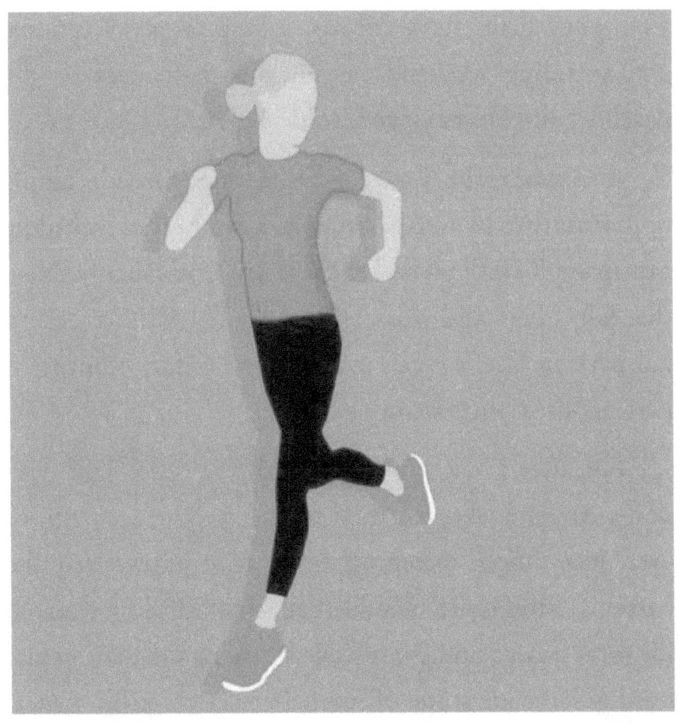

DIET & FITNESS

Helpful Hacks to get your mind in the game — and your body back in the gym.

Look at your day as a series of individual opportunities to make a healthy choice, instead of an "all or nothing" mentality where one slip up can derail you.

If your fitness routine has been less than consistent over the past few months, you're likely not alone. Summer is a unique season: longer days often consist of making after-work plans with friends, taking family vacations, and spending weekends at outdoor barbecues or the beach — not hours logged inside a gym.

And while the warm weather does provide ample opportunity to be active outdoors, a more erratic schedule can make it difficult to schedule it inconsistently. Now that fall is here and work and family obligations tend to fall back in line, we can make fitness a more consistent part of our routine again.

But after a few lax months, this is easier said than done. Anyone who has tried to lose weight, tone up, or even just simply recommit to exercise knows that the battle is often more mental than physical. So I research for some advice on how my clients overcome that mental hurdle. Here are some of my best research result mental hacks to get your mind in the game — and your body back in the gym.

Trim down your goals

Setting concrete goals is a great way to get your head back in the game and science shows that doing so does encourage behaviour change when it comes to diet and fitness. But setting the right kind of goal is key. One that is too lofty has the potential to have the opposite effect, leaving us discouraged and preventing us from sticking with it. This is why many health experts encourage us to set "SMART" goals: Specific, measurable, attainable, relevant, and time-bound.

As a personal trainer I in on the "attainable" aspect by encouraging people to make their goals more manageable. This could mean reducing your weight-loss goal, lowering the amount of produce you aim to eat each day, or shortening the amount of time you schedule at the gym. It may sound odd to aim to achieve less, but as a trainer I cites an example of one of my weight-loss clients who found success with this method: "One of my clients had a step tracker and the default setting was 10,000 steps a day. It sounds doable, but this client was consistently falling short, she would barely hit 8,000 most days. So I asked her, 'Why are you setting this goal at something you're never achieving, and then at the end of the day you feel so bad about yourself?'" and this is fact.

According to me the solution is simple: Make it attainable by going micro. "You're training your brain that you are successful. If I lower her goal to 8,000 steps, she's constantly hitting that goal, and that makes her feel confident, happy, and strong — like she can do it," she says. Once my client built a momentum of seeing that she could accomplish her goal each day, she steadily increased it and is now at 12,000 steps a day. "It took six weeks, but it's because of that instant gratification you get from seeing that goal hit by the end of the day; you see that you hit your goal or even surpassed it and that motivates you to keep going,"

Adopt a 'go with the flow attitude

"I have one client who used to get ready for a workout class and if she was five minutes late or got the wrong time for the class, she'd just go home instead of working out in the gym," says Mansour. "She said she was too embarrassed to interrupt the class and felt defeated, so she went home." (Going home often meant soothing the defeat with pizza on the couch. See: all or nothing mentality below.)

Instead of retreating home, that having more of a "go with the flow" mind-set instead of being so rigid and structured will enable you to create a Plan B (and C and D) to fall back on when things don't go as planned (which, will inevitably happen). In this client's case, a Plan B meant hopping on a treadmill for the duration of the class on the days when she is a few minutes late.

This also means being more flexible in incorporating movement throughout the day. Many of us have a rigid view of what constitutes "exercise," but the truth is that if you can't make it to the gym, there are countless ways to get that movement in elsewhere in your day. "If you live in a two-story home, go up and down the stairs for 10 minutes; have a separate bag in your car and in your office that includes headphones plus clothes and sneakers so you're prepared; if you walk your dog, commit to walking one block speed walking and then one block regular pace walking to add intervals into your nightly chore; if you're doing laundry, do 10 overhead presses then 10 squats before and after each load,"

Make skipping a workout a conscious decision

Often, deciding to skip a workout isn't a decision at all: We sleep late and don't get to the gym or we sit down to rest on the couch when we get home and time gets away from us.

As a fitness trainer I always encourages people to make this an active choice that we have control over, versus something happening to us. By making it a conscious decision, you're holding yourself accountable — and making an effort to cancel your workout plans.

"People say out of sight out of mind — the same thing with workout equipment and wardrobe," How do we keep them insight? I offers up a trick: Put your gym bag and the yoga mat on your couch, so that before you sit down to watch TV after work, you have to consciously decide to not exercise, and physically move your workout gear off the couch to sit down. Some other ideas are: sleep in your workout clothes or put them on before you leave the office so that you have to choose to take them off without exercising or leave your sneakers or gym bag sitting somewhere front and centre so you have to make the conscious choice to leave them there. Chances are when you have to exert extra effort to not exercise, you'll be more likely to follow through with your original plans.

Don't get pigeonholed into one type of workout

It's easy to fall into the hype of trendy diets and workouts, but health isn't one size fits all and what works for one person may not garner the same results for another. What works for you at one time of your life may not work at another.

"Clients come to me all the time saying they're busting their butt in the gym for weeks and months, but not seeing any results," "If something isn't working for you, try something new. Think about what your body needs. It's okay to make a change if something isn't working for you. After four weeks if you see no changes, switch to a different type of workout."

As a fitness trainer I cites one of my client who became frustrated when the workout regimen and food plan that helped her lose weight in her thirties wasn't working in her fifties. But, in her fifties she was a lot more stressed, wasn't sleeping well, was going through menopause, and was holding her weight in different areas, When she replaced kickboxing with yoga (which helped her not only tone up but lower her stress levels) she was able to lose 15 pounds.

"Instead of feeling pigeonholed into a certain workout plan, I encourage everyone to feel empowered to be the president of their workouts."

Forget the 'all or nothing' mentality – look at each day as a series of choices

"The all or nothing approach does not serve you," who says the majority of our clients suffer from this mentality. Either they start a diet or weight-loss program and are totally all in or they are totally off the wagon.

"With the holidays coming up, some people say 'I'm going to start my weight-loss goals in January' or 'I'm going to start eating healthy after the holidays' those are examples of the all or nothing mentality and that is self-sabotage," "Very successful people tend to say 'I'm all in or I'm all out.' When we look at our health in that way it sets us up to feel like we're failing if we're not hitting every single thing."

People tend to say 'I'm all in or I'm all out.' When we look at our health in that way it sets us up to feel like we're failing.

We can all relate to falling victim to this at some point: Perhaps it was eating that piece of cake at the office party that sent your diet spiralling for the rest of the day (might as well order pizza for dinner if you already slipped up, right?). Or maybe you hit snooze one too many times and missed your spin class, so you just skipped working out altogether.

To combat this, I advises my client to reframe the way we think about our health, taking it from being an overarching long-term project that we must stay on top of all of the time to being individual opportunities to make a healthy choice. "I encourage my clients to go choice by choice. In one day, you have, say, 40 decisions related to your health to make. So if you choose to work out, that's one. If you decide to work out longer than five minutes, that's another. It's choice after choice that builds on itself in that day. It's not that you have to wait until the next day to start over. It's all those individual choices."

CHAPTER – 13

How to Make Your Fitness Routine When You are Busy

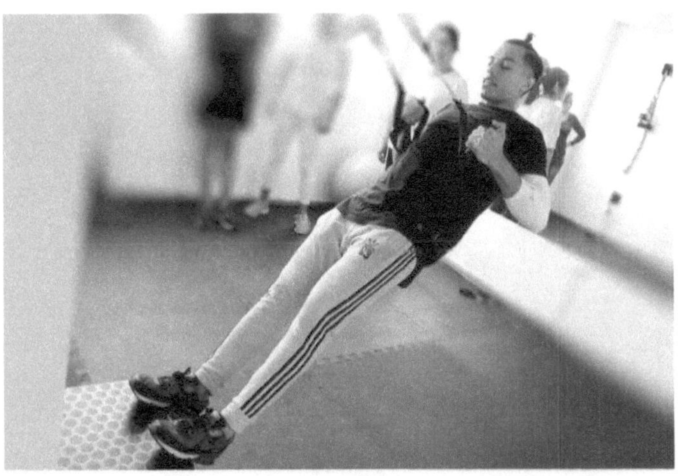

It's always better and advisable to do something rather doing nothing

TRY THESE FITNESS ROUTINES

- 10 core abs exercises that are better for your back (and body) than crunches.

- Legs exercises you can perform anywhere, anytime.

- A 10-minute functional workout you can do at home.

- 5 exercises that will strengthen your back and reduce pain.

- 15 minutes extension rope workout.

You all can check our social media platform for the above workout and can contact us anytime.

CHAPTER – 14

Psychology of Exercise

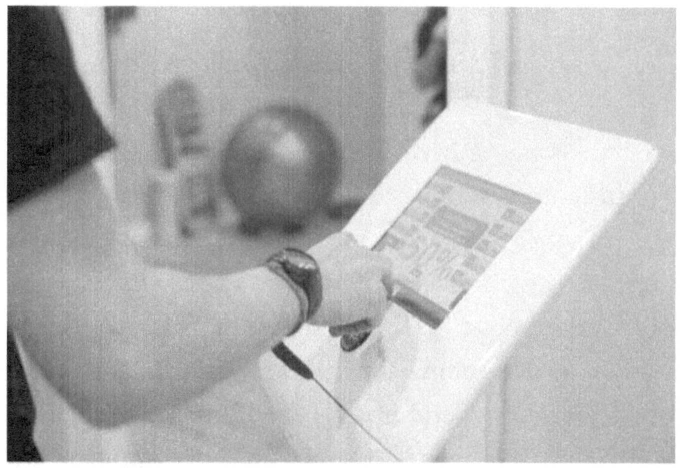

The deluge of exercise and health books in book shops and health foods in groceries is a clear indicator that people are serious about their wellbeing. People are shelling out money to buy food that contains antioxidants, monounsaturated fats, and plant compounds, swapping their sugar-enriched cereal for whole grains, all in the hope to slash their risk for heart diseases, cancer, and diabetes. Moreover, lifestyle measures are given a make-over. We now see more people in sweats armed with pedometers, jogging every morning. Gyms are no longer just home to body-building enthusiasts but also those who simply just want to lower their risk of cardiovascular diseases by sweating it out. One may even employ the services of a professional trainer. For others, an exercise physiologist would make a better partner.

An exercise physiologist is different from a personal trainer, So what does an exercise physiologist do? More precisely, what is exercise physiology?

To further define exercise physiology, it would be better to break down the terms- exercise and physiology. Exercise is any activity done that requires physical effort. For instance, walking is a form of exercise for it requires the use of legs and feet to do so. Doing any form of exercise is crucial in contributing to person wellness for it does various positive effects on one's body such as weight loss, an increase of metabolism by burning energy, staves off depression by stimulating endorphins (which sends a signal to the brain, emitting sense of control to the person), unclogs the blood vessel, thus preventing high blood pressure, high cholesterol, which in turn may lead to heart diseases.

Physiology, on the other hand, pertains to the study of functions of the living organism. It serves as the basis for studying fundamental systems. Exercise physiology, therefore, deals not just with the biological aspect of exercise but also the processes that affect the function of human organ systems (Exercise Physiology 2007).

Additionally, exercise physiology studies how exercise affects one's nutrition and energy.

It is aimed to improve one's health. For example, a person with a cardiovascular problem comes in for cardiovascular training. The exercise physiologist would then explore the person's lifestyle, conduct biological and experimental variability using heart rates, and see how the heart responds to exercise. This ensures that the treatment would target the problematic cardiovascular system.

Exercise physiology provides answers to specific questions through systematic investigation. Not a single organ system is ignored. It is like tearing apart a gadget to know and understand how each part is related, to identify how the gadget works, and be able to put them back together in case it gets broken. The body system is a complex, interconnected system that if one system is waving a red flag, the other system, would, in one way or another, get affected, like a domino effect. Engaging in exercise physiology enables treatment of the red flags while identifying possible solutions to avoid the domino effect, too.

Exercise physiology targeted at the cardiovascular system is common. Heart diseases rank number one among the cause of death in American women (Chesnutt 72). A silent killer, cardiovascular-related illnesses contribute to the death of 267,000 every year, equivalent to 43 % (72). And that is just for women alone. The danger of cardiovascular diseases is that symptoms are subtle that people usually mistake it for the occasional fatigue. Thus, it is important to increase one's cardiovascular stamina.

Cardiovascular exercises do not merely lower blood pressure and burns calories, they also enable the heart to function better. The cardiovascular system is responsible for bringing oxygen and other nutrients in the body's tissue, flushing carbon dioxide and substances to other parts of the body like the lungs and liver. In a cardiovascular system targeted exercise, six physiological aspects are considered: heart rate, stroke volume, cardiac output, blood flow, blood pressure, and blood.

The heart rate increases as the training intensify. Increasing exercise intensity leads to the attainment of the maximum heart rate. The maximum heart rate is projected using the formula 220-age. However, if the intensity remains constant, the heart rate would start becoming steady, a condition which is also known as steady-state heart rate. This happens when the cardiovascular system can meet the demands of the active tissues.

Stroke volume, or the amount of blood that is expelled per beat from the left ventricle, also increases as the training intensifies. It may reach up to 110-120ml/ beat from the average 50-70m/beat.

Another important factor that needs to be measured in the exercise physiology of the cardiovascular system is cardiac output. Cardiac output pertains to the amount of blood that the heart pumps in one minute. It is the result of the stroke volume and the heart and is computed as SV x HR.

It is also important to check the blood flow during an exercise. When the training intensifies, circulating blood shoots up to 85% of cardiac output.

The blood pressure is likewise measured before and after taking an exercise. Systolic pressure increases when the exercise intensifies. Diastolic pressure, on the other hand, roughly stays more or less the same.

Exercises cause an increase in blood volume. Experts says, a noted cardiovascular physiologist, drafted a formula in determining the rate of oxygen consumption (VO2) by computing the cardiac output (Q) and arterial-venous oxygen difference (a-v O2 diff); the resulting formula is as follows- VO2=Q x a-v O2diff.

Exercise-related measurements differ between men and women. Thus, it is important to have an exercise physiologist on hand to guide. Age is also a factor in changes in exercise physiology. A decrease in functional capacity occurs when one age.

The staggering increase of diseases around the world has put the physiology of exercise at the core. It is not enough to simply comprehend the physiological mechanisms of exercise; an exercise physiologist is also on the battlefront in promoting health and wellness in society.

While the certification is relatively new, exercise physiologists are confident that they would be recognized as healthcare professionals in the future. Exercise physiologists are working at differentiating themselves from trainers and fitness instructors. One thing that would help them achieve this goal is awareness.

If people are aware that there are licensed professionals that would not just prescribe training workouts but would also study the biological effects of in on our bodies, there is a wider opportunity for them to see these certified exercise physiologists rather than go to a gym trainer. There should not be discrimination between the two for each has his expertise. Exercise physiologists and gym trainers should not compete, though. What is important is for people to have choices in selecting how they would go into a regimen of physical activity.

CHAPTER – 15

Don't Give Up

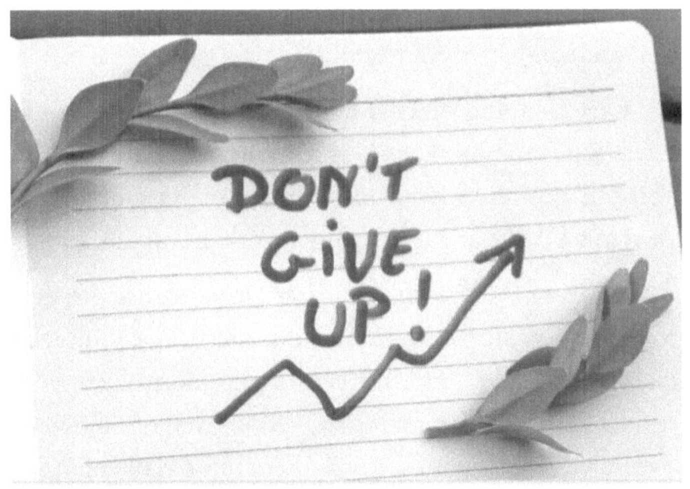

There is nothing called shortcuts in the workout, and body transformation patience is required for any workout plan.

Why people give up normally:-

You Don't Enjoy Exercise

Any exercise may feel hard at first, especially if you're just getting started. But as you become more consistent, your body gets stronger. And while enjoying exercise may seem impossible, once you've found a routine that fits your personality and lifestyle, you might find yourself looking forward to your workout.

There are many different forms of exercise, and you don't necessarily have to commit to the first one you try. Explore different forms, such as:

Group fitness: If you like social exercise, most gyms offer a variety of everything from spinning and kickboxing to circuit and strength training.

Exercised and videos: Many cable packages include Exercised, a station that offers workouts anytime you like. You can also check your local library or shop online for workout DVDs or even stream a workout on YouTube.

Work out at home: You don't have to hit the gym to get in a great workout. You can use your equipment, like hand weights, right in your living room. Even your regular chores, like raking leaves, shovelling snow, or sweeping, burn calories. Make them more challenging to up their benefit (e.g., rake small piles of leaves instead of large ones so you need to squat down to gather them more often).

Fitness apps: Downloading a variety of fitness apps on your smartphone or tablet can be like having your very own personal trainer. These apps offer ideas for workouts, ways to track your progress, and can help you stay motivated. In some cases, you can even connect and compete with others in the fitness community.

You Keep Quitting

You might start strong and with the best intentions, but before you know it, you've lost your motivation. People quit exercising for many reasons, including:

Too much too soon: If you go from no exercise at all to hitting the gym seven days a week, you're bound to feel burnt out. Instead, ease into a new routine.

Confusion: Do your research. Find out more about the machines at the gym and learn a little basic anatomy so you can target your exercises to your goals. If you go in without a plan, you're more likely to choose random exercises or complete them sporadically. Most gyms offer how-to tours of their facilities.

Boredom: Some people love treadmills or stationary bikes, but others find walking or pedalling to nowhere get old fast. If you're quickly getting bored with the exercises you've chosen, they may not be a good fit. Find something that holds your interest for the long haul or that offers enough variety to keep your workout from feeling stale.

Soreness: When you're just starting, soreness is to be expected. However, you should still be able to function. If you're so exhausted after your workout that you can't lift your head off the pillow or you get an injury while exercising, you're not likely to feel motivated to get back to it once you're feeling better.

If you're tempted to quit, take it as a sign that it's time to change up your routine.

Work with a trainer: An experienced trainer can turn a lacklustre workout into an effective and challenging routine.

Change your workouts: Try different types of training to keep things interesting, such as circuit training, high-intensity interval training, and kettlebells. Be sure to balance strength with cardio workouts. This also helps you avoid plateaus.

Avoid skipping: If you want to skip out on the gym, there's probably a reason. Think about what it is and if it's something you really can overcome.

You Can't Afford a Gym Membership

There's no reason you have to join a gym to exercise, but if you're determined to leave the house to work out, there are more affordable options such as the local community centres. To save money on workouts, you can also try:

- Walking or running: All you need is a good pair of shoes for this simple, accessible workout.

- Buy multi-use equipment: An exercise ball can be used for core work, weight training, and even cardio. Dumbbells are usually inexpensive and can be used for the entire body.

- Workout at home: If you need ideas, look to videos for inspiration. You can also make up your routines—just put on some music and get moving.

- Find free resources: The Internet is a great source

for workouts and weight loss programs, and your library is an excellent resource for trying workout videos or finding books about exercise.

- Try no equipment workouts: You can get a great workout without any equipment by using your body weight.

You're Not Seeing Changes in Your Body

If you're not losing weight as fast as you hoped or getting sculpted abs, the frustration might make you want to throw in the towel. Remember: You don't put weight on or become deconditioned overnight. Likewise, you can't lose weight or rebuild your strength overnight either.

Getting started is the first step toward reaching your fitness goals. Give your body time to react.

Make sure you've set realistic fitness goals and understand how weight loss works. In the meantime, stay focused on the many other benefits of physical activity, such as reducing stress and improving posture.

You Don't Know How to Exercise

Being an exercise beginner can be overwhelming (and even intimidating). There are many different types of exercise you can try. Some will work for you and others might not. Figuring that out for yourself can be challenging. The good news is, there are plenty of resources out there to help.

If you're part of a gym or fitness centre, consider working with a personal trainer. If you're working out at home or on a budget, try getting started with an online fitness program.

You Have Childcare Responsibilities:-

With school and after-school activities and sports, kids and teens can have schedules as busy as their parents. Just because you have carpool duty or need to make sure your teen gets to practice on time doesn't mean you have to neglect your own fitness goals.2 In fact, exercise can be a great activity for the whole family. Making time for a workout doesn't just benefit your health; it also sets a good example for your kids.

Exercising with kids requires planning, but it's not impossible. If you look to your community, you'll likely find some good resources.

- Join a health club or gym with a day-care centre.

- Put on an exercise video when the kids are napping or you're waiting for dinner to cook.

- If they're old enough, invite your kids to be part of your routine. Show them how to lift small weights, have them count your repetitions, or take them along on your daily walk.

- Find family-friendly activities in your community. If you'd enjoy coaching or mentoring, see if there are opportunities involved with your child's sports team.

- Rethink exercise: Challenging kids to a running

race or playing an animated game of tag can burn calories too.

You're Too Stressed

Being stressed can make everything more difficult to face—workouts included. At the same time, waiting to feel like you want to exercise can backfire. Motivation is something you have to work at every day. Here are a few tips you can try:

- Set reasonable weight loss goals and remind yourself of them every day.

- Each time you reach a goal, whether it's completing your workouts for the week, losing weight, or feeling more energized, reward yourself. Go for a massage, put together a new workout playlist, buy new running shoes, or spend a quiet night at home curled up with a good book.

- Talk with others about their goals and how they stay motivated. If you aren't part of a gym or class, join some message boards or social media groups.

- Focus on how you feel rather than the numbers on the scale or what you see in the mirror, at least in the beginning. If weight loss is slow or you aren't seeing changes in your body as soon as you'd hoped, it can be discouraging. But there are other benefits to working out, such as better balance and more energy that you might be overlooking.

You're tired and sore

Exercise can be uncomfortable, especially in the beginning when you're trying to find your stride. Once your body adapts, it starts to get easier. Still, even experienced fitness gurus experience some soreness after a hard workout.

If your workout is truly painful, you may need to try something else to avoid injury. If the soreness is just the result of your body getting used to moving more, here are some things you can try:

- Ease into it: Start with a few days of moderate cardio (like walking) and basic strength workouts to build endurance and strength.

- Stay in your target heart rate zone: You should be able to carry on a conversation if you're working at a moderate intensity.

- Start with light weights: With weight training, an effort is needed to build lean body tissue. When you're just starting, any weight you lift is going to require effort. In the early days, focus more on maintaining good form. Then increase your weight once you've mastered the exercise.

- Take extra rest days: If you're more sore or exhausted than usual, or haven't changed up your routine, take it as a sign your body needs an extra rest day to repair and recover.

You Can't Commit

When you only think about exercise in the long term ("I have to do this forever!"), it can be overwhelming. Keep in mind that you don't have to change everything in your life all at once, and not all the changes you make have to happen overnight. If you're having trouble sticking to your workout routine, try to:

- Start with small goals: It's easier to stick with a workout when your goals start small. Try challenging yourself to walk an extra 10 minutes each day or get up early for a short yoga workout.

- Plan ahead: Schedule your workouts and prepare for them ahead of time so you're not tempted to skip them.

- Make exercise a priority: Ask yourself if a fitness routine is truly important to you or if you just want it to be. Making exercise a priority takes commitment, and commitment takes motivation. Figure out what your goals are, but keep them realistic.

- Don't focus only on weight loss: If your only goal is weight loss, it can be hard to stick to a routine if you don't see results right away. While you don't want to lose sight of your long-term goals, try giving some of your attention and focus to the other benefits of exercise.

You Don't Have Time

When you're looking at your to-do list, it might feel like you just don't have time to exercise. But exercise doesn't need to take a lot of time to be effective. And, if you look more closely at how you spend your time, you might realize you've got more of it to carve out than you thought.

- Put your workout on your schedule. Keep a calendar of your workouts so you can track your progress and stay motivated.

- Just because you can't find a 30-minute slot of time during your day for a workout doesn't mean you can't work out at all. Try breaking your activity up into 10- or 15-minute segments. Research has shown that split workouts are just as effective as continuous workouts.

- Get up a few minutes early and take a brisk walk, use part of your lunch break for a stretch, or take the dog out for a romp after work. Even small changes, like parking at the far side of the lot or taking the stairs when possible, add up over time.

- Remember: Exercise generates energy. The more energy you have, the more you'll get done each day.

So before quitting please think about why you have started. And to escape this situation you need to set goals have to find a reason or a proper way or manner to set a goal. Setting your goals is a bold play for your best life. Setting your goals is an act of heroism because you are reaching for the potential that has been invested in you.

Setting Goals

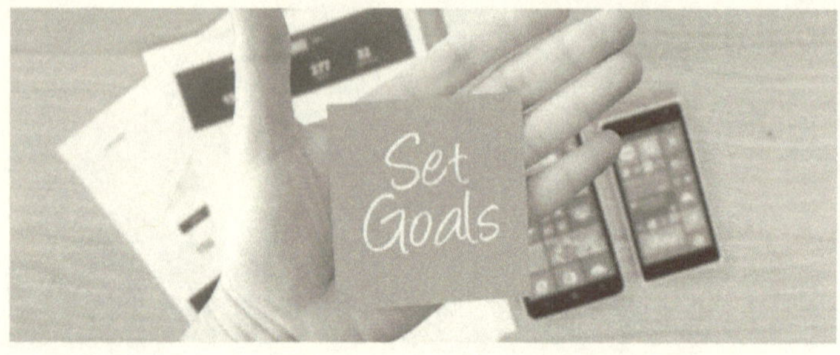

Experts say: - there are six big reasons for you to set goals: -

Focus, Growth, Intentionality, Measurements, Alignment, and Inspiration.

Focus:-

1. Focus on what you should eat. Too often, diets focus on what you shouldn't eat, not what you should eat. Instead of concentrating on what to cut out, try building a meal plan from the ground up that fills your day with healthy, balanced meals. One of the best ways to keep yourself on track is to build a detailed meal plan in advance so that you won't draw a blank when you get hungry.

2. Choose real food. While we're on the topic of what you should be eating, a good general rule to follow is to choose real food – food that's found in nature – over heavily processed options that are full of chemicals and additives. Yes, you can probably lose weight with low-calorie options no matter how many unpronounceable words are in the ingredients list, but that doesn't make them healthy. Ditch the weight-loss shakes and bars and opt for fruits and vegetables that will keep you slim while giving you the nutrients you need to keep your body functioning at its best.

3. Drink more water. Water packs a dual punch! It's healthy and helps you lose weight. Not only does water help flush the toxins from your body, but studies show that drinking more water can significantly boost your metabolism. It also helps fill you up so that you don't feel the need to eat as much. Cut out the empty calories of soda and other sweet drinks and replace them with life-sustaining H2O.

4. Listen to your body. It may seem obvious, but one of the best ways to lose weight is also one of the simplest: Only eat when you're hungry. Next time you reach for the fridge, take a minute to consider whether you're really in need of nourishment or whether you're just trying to pass the time. Keeping in tune with your body's true needs will

keep you on course – not only to weight loss but also to overall health.

5.   Use food as an opportunity to practice being mindful and grateful. As important as it is to take care of your body, it's also important to take care of your mind. Research shows that actively practicing gratitude is one of the best ways to increase happiness levels. That's a great reason to start thinking more mindfully about the food you're eating and to use mealtimes as a chance to express gratefulness. Whether that involves saying grace out loud with your family or just taking a moment to appreciate the food on the table in front of you, a less absent-minded approach to eating can bring great rewards.

6.   Cheat when you need to, but don't let it turn into a pattern. Whether it's having a slice of wedding cake or enjoying a mixed drink during a night out with friends, we get it. Sometimes you need to "cheat," and in the right context cheating can even be healthy – for your mental health, that is. Do it, don't dwell on it, and don't let that nagging voice in your head convince you that there's no turning back.

7.   Discover a form of exercise that energizes you. A good exercise regimen should tire you out, but it shouldn't feel like torture. If you're running on the treadmill with your eyes glued to the calorie-

burning counter, it might be time to reconsider your approach to working out. If you don't love cardio? Try strength training. Feeling left behind at the yoga studio? Try a Zumba class. Finding your fit will make you more likely to keep up your exercise routine over the long term.

8. Power your body with essential nutrients. If you have any particular nutritional concerns, consider taking natural, food-based supplements to fill in any gaps. Consult a professional to learn more about how supplements can ensure that you get the vitamins and minerals you need.

9. Don't just copy what worked for others. Just because you've heard that a particular fad diet worked for someone else doesn't mean that it will work for you. You're an individual, and you need an individual weight loss plan. If you want to take a more formal approach to wellness and weight loss, choose a company like NAGA Fitess.com that will develop a personalized plan tailored to your circumstances.

Growth:-

Growth is a continuous process it is defined as an irreversible constant increase in the size of an organ or even an individual cell. Put differently, growth is the most fundamental characteristic of living bodies accompanied by various metabolic processes that take place at the cost of energy. The processes can be anabolic or catabolic. When it comes to plants, the seeds germinate, develop into a seedling, and acquires a shape of an adult plant are discrete stages of growth and the growth of Plants is indefinite.

In the Biological term, there's a minute difference between the terms growth and development. These words describe a separate set of events in an organism or plant.

Growth refers to the increase in mass and size of a body.

Development is the process where a particular organism, not only grows physically but acquires mental and physiological growth as well. In weight loss and body transformation, it is considered as a continuous process a journey. To go on.

Intentionality:-

In philosophy, intentionality is the power of minds and mental states to be about, to represent, or to stand for, things, properties, and states of affairs. To say of an individual's mental states that they have intentionality is to say that they are mental representations or that they have contents. Furthermore, to the extent that a speaker utters words from some natural language or draws pictures or symbols from a formal language to convey to others the contents of her mental states, these artefacts used by a speaker too have contents or intentionality. 'Intentionality' is a philosopher's word: ever since it was introduced into philosophy by Franz Brentano in the last quarter of the nineteenth century, it has been used to refer to the puzzles of representation, all of which lie at the interface between the philosophy of mind and the philosophy of language. A picture of a dog, a proper name, the common noun 'dog' or the concept expressed by the word can mean, represent, or stand for, one or several hairy barking creatures. A complete thought, a full sentence, or a picture can stand for or describe a state of affairs. How could some of the represented things (e.g., dinosaurs) be arbitrarily remote in space and time from the representation (e.g., human thought or utterance about dinosaurs tokened in 2018), while others (e.g., numbers) may not even be in space and time at all? How could some representations (e.g., direct quotations such as 'dinosaur') even stand for themselves? How does a complex representation (e.g., a complete thought or a full-sentence) inherit its meaning or content from the meanings or contents of its constituents? How should one construe the relationship between the iconic content of pictorial representations and the conceptual content of proposition-like representations (thoughts and utterances)? How should one understand the relation between the content of an individual's mental state and the meanings of external symbols used by the individual to express her internal mental states? Are representations of the world part of the world they represent? Do all of an individual's mental states have intentionality or only some of them?

In body transformation context it comes mental states of you to achieve your goal, how much you are commuted for your goal.

Measurements:-

This is the most important part after focus and intention to be cleared measurement is required to measure your success in the given timeline, how much you have achieved, and in what quantity. Measurement is required to measure the journey and it is required to measure or calculate the future timeline of success, but in bodyweight transformation and weight loss we should measure but we should more focus on the continuity part, not the result part if somehow result from not come as per our expectations then their negativity occurs.

- A measurement is the action of measuring something or some amount of stuff.

- So it is important to measure certain things right, distance, time, and accuracy are all great things to measure.

- By measuring these things or in other words, by taking these measurements we can better understand the world around us.

- Measurements can also allow us to make decisions based on the outcome of the measurement.

- By this reasoning measurements are extremely important because they shape the way we think and interact every day.

Alignment:-

Alignment means arranging everything properly including your workout diet sleep rest and everything that you require in body transformation. And proper posture and form also play an important role in body transformation.

Taking the time to align your body with the correct form prevents injury. It also helps you balance your muscle groups for long-term postural benefits.

The body and the muscles and joints of the bodywork best when the body is in a certain alignment whole moving. These ideal positions help the muscles and joints to produce and reduce force in the best manner. The ability to optimally produce and reduce force is what minimizes the risk of injury. The best to ensure proper body alignment is to eliminate any muscle imbalances by identifying them and getting rid of them. Muscular imbalances can be identified using movement assessments like the overhead squat. During movement, the body's joints will move based on what muscles are tight, weak, or not working optimally. Once you identify muscle imbalances, strengthen weakened muscles, lengthen tight ones and this will improve posture and help train good form. If you want to learn how to identify muscle imbalances consult a personal trainer experienced in performing muscle imbalance tests.

Inspiration Motivation:-

I'm so excited to be here today, talking to you all about losing weight by choosing a healthy lifestyle. You might ask, "How do you know what I'm going through?"

One year ago i was 90 kg. That January I made a resolution to do whatever I needed to do to become healthy. I told my friends, "I'm going to lose weight. When you see me this time next year, you will see a different woman."

People wished me well, but I'm sure they had their doubts. After all, I had tried fad diets before. Sometimes I lost weight, but I always ended up gaining it all back plus some. This time was different.

I made the lifestyle changes that were needed to get me to the healthy weight of 65 kg today. I'm here today to tell you that you can do it too. You can lose weight, keep it off, and live a healthier life.

I truly believe that the biggest factor in developing a healthy eating lifestyle is a positive, determined frame of mind. Diet plans I tried in the past didn't work, but to be honest I never really expected them to work.

The difference for me came from telling myself, "This is it. You can do it. You WILL do it." I didn't focus mainly on weight loss but on empowering myself to set goals and then meet them.

It is important to think positive thoughts about yourself and your journey to a healthy lifestyle. You may face hard times during your transition. The key is to stay focused on your goals and you will always reach them. Like Ralph Marston has said, "Your goals, minus your doubts, equal your reality."

Once I knew I was going to become healthier and lose weight, the next thing I did was throw away all the junk food in my house.

I don't know about you, but I knew if the food was in there, I was going to eat it. Anytime I went shopping after that only healthy foods made it into the house. I didn't starve myself. I like to eat too much for that!

It was all about learning a new way to eat. Every day I would fill up on vegetables, fruit, and lean meats. I encourage everyone here today to do a quick inventory of your pantry when you get home. Are these the foods that can help you become the healthy person you want to be?

My next step was to start exercising. At first, it was difficult for me. I would get out of breath just getting ready to exercise! Did I let that stop me? No!

Every day I did as much as I could. I got off the couch and spent time outside. I parked wherever there was a spot instead of driving around waiting for the closest one. Gradually, I was able to exercise more and more until I reached the point where I was able to jog 5km every day.

This isn't a diet so there is no ending point. It is all about living every day, making the right choices for my health. That is what has helped me to lose almost more then 20 kg in 4 months. That is what has made it possible for me to do the things I want to do because I have the energy.

I decide to be healthy every day when I wake up. You can make that same decision. I believe in you. Believe in yourself, lose weight, and live the healthy lifestyle you have always wanted.

CHAPTER – 17

What Is the Difference Between Happiness and Pleasure

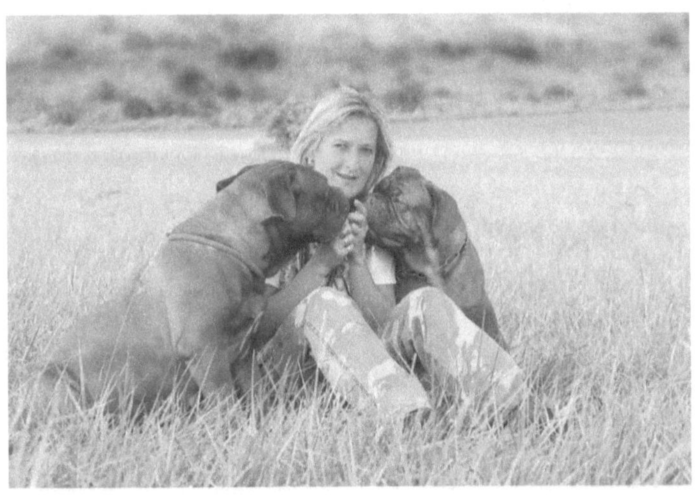

Pleasure is a state, in which you feel good and enjoy what you are doing. Pleasure is usually caused by external stimuli and often involves the five senses. Here are a few examples:

- We enjoy the warmth under the blanket on cold winter days.

- We experience a sensation of pleasure when we eat a delicious slice of cake.

- We get pleasure when we listen to pleasant music.

- We experience pleasure when we do something we love doing.

- We also derive pleasure from reading a book and from daydreaming.

- We get pleasure from the smell and taste of good food, from a pleasant breeze on a warm day, or the sight of a beautiful person.

Pleasure often does not last long, since soon the attention moves to other matters. We enjoy the pleasure we experience, but after a while, we either lose interest or seek something else. For example, you might eat a piece of chocolate and enjoy it, but after a few pieces of chocolate, you feel you cannot eat anymore.

Sometimes, too much of something stops being enjoyable.

Often, we have other things we need to do, like work, cleaning the house, driving somewhere, fixing something, or carrying tasks or chores we do not like. Then, we have to stop doing the activity that is giving us pleasure and do other things.

- When you eat some delicious food you derive pleasure from it, but the pleasure doesn't last for long, since you cannot go on eating indefinitely. Sometimes after you finish eating the food on your plate, the sensation of pleasure wears off.

- You may enjoy watching a movie, but the movie lasts for a certain amount of minutes, and when you return to your everyday reality.

- When you read a book that you enjoy reading, ultimately, you arrive at the last page. The memory of the book might linger on, but then you look for something else to do.

As you see, all pleasure is time-limited.

What Is Happiness and How It Differs from Pleasure

Pleasure is emotional in nature, and often depends on the five senses, while happiness is different, it is an inner sensation. In pleasure the emotions and feelings are active. In a state of happiness, there is calmness and peace.

Happiness might be triggered by events or external factors, but it does not depend on them. It is a sensation of inner calmness and satisfaction.

Though happiness is similar to pleasure in some respects, yet it is different.

When do you feel happy? You usually feel happy when a problem has been solved, when you receive good news when a goal has been accomplished when you earn a great sum of money, or when you are deeply in love.

For a few moments, you feel happy. What do you feel?

You feel free, blissful, as if the sun is shining on you, and you have no worries and nothing is bothering you. It is a state of exhilaration and peace. For a few moments, you feel as if a burden has been lifted, and you feel no fears or doubts, and don't think about the next thing you are going to do.

For few moments, there are no thoughts and there is no time. These are moments of peace and happiness. You experience a deep feeling of relief, without any thinking, doubts, or expectations. For a moment your mind is empty.

In this "empty state", happiness arises. It usually does not stay for long, since you cannot stay in this state for long. Your mind is not trained to be peaceful, and all the thoughts, desires, doubts, fears, or expectations rise back again, hiding the calmness you experienced just a moment ago.

As you see, happiness is a state of inner peace and inner calmness.

Everyone seeks happiness when actually, the search is for inner peace and freedom from nonstop thinking.

Happiness and inner peace come from the same source, from within. Through training, one can reach a state when happiness and peace are experienced more and more often.

The more you can free your mind from the compulsion of thinking nonstop, moving from one thought to another, without any rest, the more you will be able to enjoy inner peace and happiness.

As you see, though pleasure and happiness bring joy and a good feeling, they are not the same thing.

We need and enjoy both pleasure and happiness, and while pleasure often has to do with physical sensations, happiness is more an inner sensation that is associated with inner peace and mental and emotional calmness.

Instead of waiting for external events to trigger happiness, you can bring it from inside you. Since inner peace has much to do with a state of happiness, the more peaceful your mind is, the more happiness you can enjoy.

When you can make your mind peaceful, you enjoy more happiness.

CHAPTER – 18

Living with Dying Daily Thought

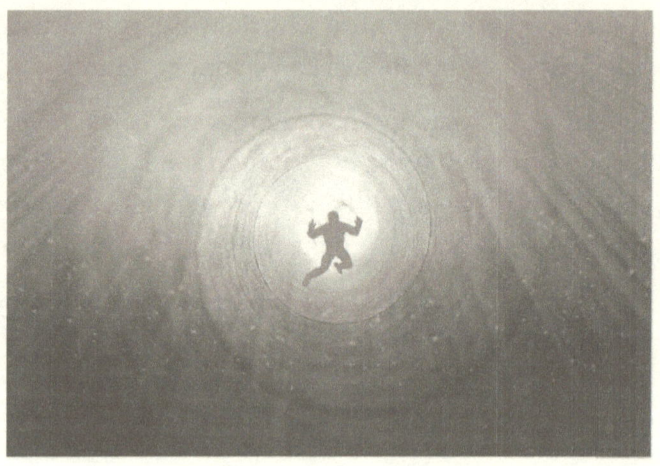

Dying Daily thoughts lead you to a happy and more valued life.

"Live as if you were to die tomorrow. Learn as if you were to live forever"

This is one of the most inspirational from Gandhi that can change one's life. The meaning behind this quote is don't be afraid to live life and try something new, let life be the reason you are living. Gandhi points out that life is something you live to the fullness and learn throughout it. Being afraid to live and learn in life is not something a person should be doing. "Live as if you were to die tomorrow." pushes people to do things in life they always wanted to do because their life is almost up and "Learn as if you were to live forever." learning since you can live forever is the most important in life if you decide to live forever. Learning is not something you get bored of, rather it is something you take in. Gandhi chooses the words "die tomorrow" and "live forever" to allow people to pretend there is no tomorrow and that you should do what you wanted in life and living forever is the opportunity to learn throughout the years you live. You will never run out of things to learn if you were to live forever.

Live as if you will die tomorrow:

This is a great line. Many people live every single day with so many regrets, depression, and stress. They all forget to live. Living is not only breathing. Living is enjoying the little things in your life. Living is making every breath count. Living is to prove to God that he did the right thing by sending you into this world. This is living. And we are doing just the opposite. We should live as if today is the last day on earth. Do what you want to do. Just take it out of your mind what people will think. You do because you want to do. This is the meaning of living like it will be our last day.

Learn as if you will live forever

It is associated with learning. It means to learn everything that you wanted to. Learn those things which give you pleasure. Learn those things which don't stand out as a source of stress for you. Many of us don't learn or don't open our minds to new ideas just because of what others will think. Why we think that people will think negatively. Why don't we think that people can also think positive thoughts? When you try a new thing, people will think that you are on the verge of becoming extraordinary. So, stop living like an old book. Open your mind to update to the new version.

CHAPTER – 19

Vision for Your Transformation

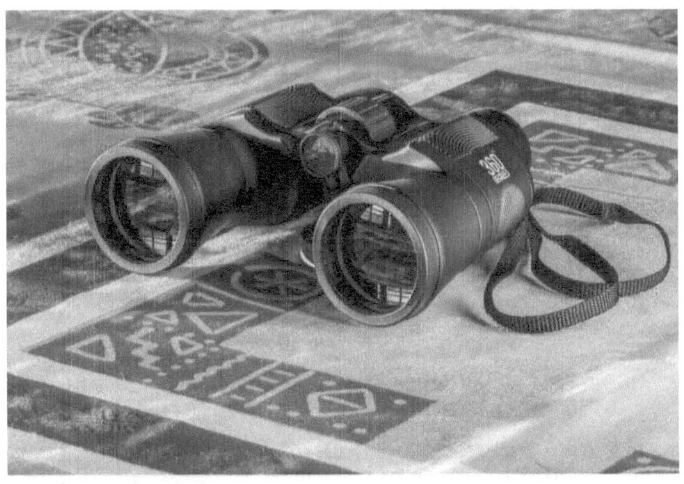

Make A vision board for your transformation journey:-

If weight loss is on your mind and you're on the hunt for motivational tips and tools that will keep you accountable to your goals, a weight loss vision board may be just the thing you need. While we all know that healthy eating, regular exercise, quality sleep, and ample water intake can all help us shed unwanted pounds, not everyone has the internal motivation and discipline needed to adopt new habits and maintain them over time. If this sounds like you, keep reading for tips and ideas to help you create a weight loss vision board that will inspire you to embrace change and keep you moving forward when you feel like giving up.

What is a Vision Board?

Also known as a 'dream board', a vision board is a visual representation of your goals. It's a collage of pictures, magazine clippings, words, affirmations, and quotes that help bring your dreams to life, serving as a daily reminder and motivator to pursue the things that move your life forward instead of remaining stagnant. Rather than focusing on your faults and failures, etc., a vision board is thought to encourage you to shift your energy towards becoming a higher version of yourself. When practiced correctly, a vision board can help you overcome self-limiting beliefs and shift your mind-set, allowing you to achieve great things in life!

What Should You Include On Your Weight Loss Vision Board?

While creating a vision board may sound therapeutic to someone who enjoys crafting, it may feel silly and overwhelming to those who aren't creatively inclined. If this sounds like you, don't allow your lack of creativity to hold you back! A vision board doesn't have to be a work of art – you can make it as simple or complex as you want to.

We dig more into the science of creating a vision board for weight loss below, but if you're looking for a high-level overview of the kinds of things you should include on your vision board, here are some ideas:

- Your big, fat, hairy, audacious goal

- Smaller, short-term goals that will help keep you accountable

- Photos and/or images that bring your goal to life

- Words and affirmations to keep you motivated when roadblocks present themselves

- Inspirational quotes to help you on days you feel like quitting

- Lists of specific action items to help you reach your goals

- Checklists to help you track your progress over time

Vision Board Supplies to Invest In

Before you start to create a vision board, you will need a few supplies. Remember that you can make this project as simple or creative as you would like to, so the amount of supplies you'll require depends on how crafty you're feeling.

- Poster board, bulletin board, or corkboard to display your items

- Tape, glue, and/or push pins to stick items to your board

- Construction paper to write words, affirmations, quotes, etc.

- Markers

- Scissors

- A selection of magazines, preferably about the topic of your vision board

- Motivational quote cards

- Poster board cut out shapes

- Quote chips

- Gel pens

How to Create a Weight Loss Vision Board?

Now that you know what a vision board is and have the supplies you need to create your own, it's time to get to work, which can feel a tad overwhelming. How do you get started? Should you have one goal or many? What kinds of pictures and graphics should you include? Where can you find words, affirmations, and quotes to inspire you? Should you include checklists? There are so many things to consider, but rest assured there is no right way to create a vision board. You can make this as simple or detailed as you want — as long as it motivates you, that's all that matters! If you're trying to create a weight loss vision board, here are some tips and ideas to get you started and help you get the most out of the process.

1. DEFINE YOUR GOAL(S)

If you're looking for weight loss vision board ideas, you most likely have a target weight in mind, but I urge you to go above and beyond the numbers on your bathroom scale. Ask yourself questions like:

- Why do I want to lose weight?

- How will I feel when I reach my goal?

- How will I look when I reach my goal?

- How will others describe me when I reach my goal?

- How will my life change when I reach my goal?

Try to envision the person you aspire to be. Is she strong? Does she have more energy? Is she an inspiration to her friends and family? Does she run marathons or compete in CrossFit competitions? You get the idea…

2. LOOK FOR PICTURES/IMAGES THAT REPRESENT YOUR GOAL

Once you've visualized this new version of yourself, look for pictures and images that help bring that vision to life. This could be a photo of a celebrity you admire, a photo of yourself when you were in better shape, or you can superimpose your head on the body of a fitness professional you aspire to become. Whichever way you choose to approach this, the idea is to create an image of the future YOU to include on your weight loss vision board, giving you something to look to for motivation when you feel like giving up.

3. CREATE A ROADMAP

Creating a vision board for weight loss goes above and beyond superimposing your face onto a photo of a fitness model. While it's great to have a visual of what you want your future self to look like, you need to create a roadmap to help you get there.

If you're creating a weight loss vision board, your road map should include short-term goals that will help you reach your overarching goal. Healthy eating, regular physical activity, drinking more water, and sleep are all examples of smaller goals you can add to your weight loss road map. Keep in mind that it can be very overwhelming (and unrealistic) to adopt multiple new habits at once, so consider creating a plan that focuses on one new goal every 1-3 months.

4. TRACK YOUR PROGRESS

Another key element to a successful weight loss vision board is progress tracking. Whether you choose to add a tracking sheet directly onto your vision board or opt to create a separate tracking spreadsheet, it's important to do regular check-ins to evaluate your progress. This can be especially helpful for weight loss as the scale only tells part of your story – measurements, pictures, the way your clothes fit, and your mood are all important factors in your journey.

5. IDENTIFY OBSTACLES THAT MAY SET YOU BACK

While creating your weight loss vision board, it can be extremely helpful to identify obstacles that might set you back along the way. Self-doubt, stress, social events, travel, and unsupportive family and friends are all examples of things that can derail your progress, but if you take the time to plan and put together a plan of action, you'll be better equipped to deal with these challenges head-on. This leads me to my next tip…

6. CURATE WORDS, AFFIRMATIONS & QUOTES

Once you've identified all of the obstacles that can and will crop up in your weight loss journey, spend some time searching for words, affirmations, and/or quotes that can help you overcome negative, self-sabotaging thoughts and replace them with positive, self-affirming beliefs. Words like STRONG, POWERFUL, WORTHY, CAPABLE, RESILIENT, ENOUGH, and BEAUTIFUL come to mind, I'm linking to my favourite motivational weight loss quotes HERE, and I've highlighted my favas below!

'Excuses don't burn calories.'

'Don't wish for it. Work for it.'

'If you're tired of starting over, stop giving up.'

'Be stronger than your excuse.'—Nike Slogan

'If it doesn't challenge you, it doesn't change you.'

'Do it because they said you couldn't.'

7. BRING IT ALL TOGETHER

Once you've identified your short-term and long-term goals, found photos, and images that represent your vision, created a roadmap and figured out how you'll track your progress, identified potential roadblocks, and written out your favourite words, affirmations, and quotes, it's time to pull it all together and personalize your weight loss vision board. Keep it simple and minimalistic, or get loud and creative – whatever works best for you and your personality!

8. PUT IT INTO PRACTICE

Once your weight loss vision board is complete, the display is somewhere prominent, like your desk, nightstand, kitchen counter, or closet to ensure you see it every single day. Refer to it when obstacles pop up and you feel your motivation slipping, and set a daily/weekly reminder on your phone to check in with your goals, track your progress, etc.

9. UPDATE YOUR VISION BOARD REGULARLY

My final tip for creating a successful weight loss vision board is to make sure you're updating it periodically. If you feel overwhelmed and discouraged by the magnitude of your original goals, go back and make adjustments. If you've identified new habits you feel would be helpful, add them. If you heard a new affirmation or quote that lights a fire under your booty, stick it on!

If you're trying to create a weight loss vision board to get you closer to your goals, I hope the tips and ideas in this post prove useful to you. Don't be afraid to set big goals, but be careful to create a realistic roadmap that will get you from where you are now to the version of yourself you hope to become. Track your progress, anticipate roadblocks, and adjust your sails when you need to!

CHAPTER – 20

Self Belief

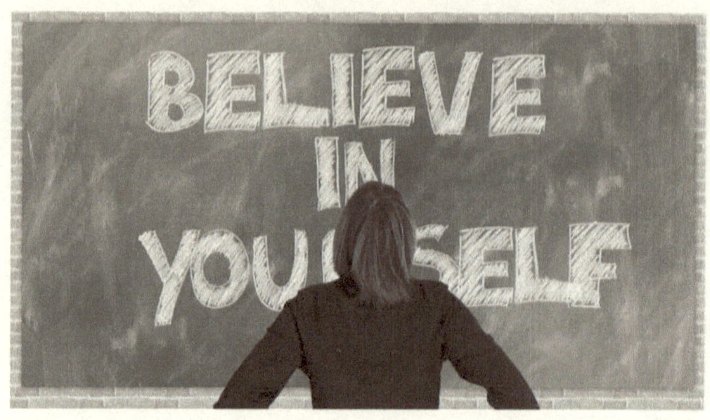

Why Self-Belief Is Important to Reach Your Full Potential

The Dalai Lama once said, "With the realization of one's potential and self-confidence in one's ability one can build a better world." In both my personal and professional life, I strive to remember that quote when the going gets tough, and both circumstances, other people, and situations conspire to undermine my confidence and fill.

The Dalai Lama once said, "With the realization of one's potential and self-confidence in one's ability one can build a better world."

In both my personal and professional life, I strive to remember that quote when the going gets tough, and both circumstances, other people, and situations conspire to undermine my confidence and fill me with the toxic neurosis of self-doubt.

Everyone needs to believe in something, and I think if you don't believe in yourself, how can you inspire others? How can you realize your ambitions? How can you fulfil your dreams, and how can you reach your full potential?

Self-belief is the source of all positivity. If you believe in yourself and what you are doing, it's contagious. Those around you will pick up on the vibe and seek to emulate your focused and driven mind-set—because a confident person is a person who gets things done. Self-belief is almost like a superpower. It can overcome any obstacle, knock down any door, and solve any problem. It's the rock I cling to which can weather any storm and the one game-changer which you need in your locker.

When you have faith in yourself, you'll be surprised at your capabilities. The great news is, only you and you alone have the power and the key to unlock your true potential and transform your life. With a little self-belief, big things can happen. Here's how:

Self-Belief and the Power of Creativity

A creative mind can become crippled with anxiety and doubt and unable to think outside of the box. When you lack confidence, everything seems like an uphill struggle. Everyday problems can loom large and appear insurmountable. Self-belief makes you relax, feel more capable, and you can see things with crystal-clear clarity. In such situations, you're able to perceive not just one but a myriad of solutions to the problem at hand.

Self-Belief and Inspiring Others

Self-belief gives off an intoxicating aura. It both enchants and captivates others. When you believe in a person, it's because they believe in themselves and their motivation. A confident individual is an inspiring individual who leads by example. Your self-belief can bring out the best in others and help them perform because they've seen first-hand the potential it unlocks.

Self-Belief and Direct Action

A person who believes in themselves doesn't hesitate or sit on the fence when it comes to making a call and follow-through. You would be surprised how many missed opportunities happen because people spend too much time debating instead of doing. It all comes down to a lack of confidence. More importantly, in business as in life, you need to prepare for setbacks and be patient if you are to achieve your goals. Without the persistence and tenacity of self-belief and the confidence you are doing the right thing and are on the right path, long-term ambitions are all but impossible.

Self-Belief and Personal Development

If a person is to realize their true potential, they need to continue to develop and evolve. Neither is possible if you don't believe in yourself. Self-belief allows room for you to make mistakes, tempered with the knowledge that it's all part of a grand learning curve and not the end of the world. And here's the thing, to build self-belief, you need to challenge yourself, and when you challenge yourself, things don't always go as planned, but there are always lessons to learn.

Self-Belief and Success

Self-belief unlocks your true potential, and this, in turn, ushers in an enormous amount of success. The two go together. Think about it. When was the last time you saw a successful person who lacked confidence? A confident person doesn't compare themselves to others, knows what they are capable of, is willing to learn, and is not afraid to dream big. "If you hear a voice within say, 'you cannot paint,' then by all means paint, and that voice will be silenced."

In other words, believe in yourself, and good things will happen.

CHAPTER – 21

Body Transformation Starts with the Mind

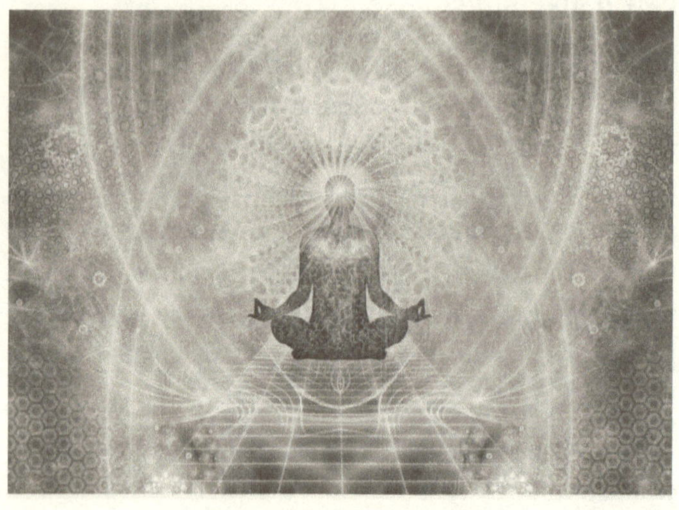

I spent few years of my life searching for the one piece of magic that would turn me into a thin, lean person. Was it cutting out carbs? Going on an incredibly low-calorie diet? Paleo? Vegan? I can honestly say I tried it all.

And each time, regardless of what plan I went on, I lost weight. But I would eventually gain it back—and sometimes more. This led to years to "weight cycling" which is not only frustrating and discouraging but has also been shown in research to be very damaging to health.

Why weren't any of these plans sustainable?

After years of beating myself up over my failed weight loss, I realized that beating myself up was probably not the way to go about it. It occurred to me that if I wanted lasting change, I needed a new way of thinking about weight loss.

You see, it wasn't the fact that I hadn't found the perfect diet; it was the mind-set that accompanied each diet that kept me from reaching my goals in the long term. To buy into the diet mind-set that motivated me to go to extremes in my eating, I had to buy into some pretty painful beliefs about myself:

I believed that I couldn't be happy unless I was thin

You see this all the time in weight loss marketing; an overweight "before" picture with ragged clothes, unwashed hair, and a pitiful frown. Then, a stunningly gorgeous "after" picture, with not only smaller clothes and a smaller waist, but also incredible hair, airbrushed skin, perfectly manicured nails, and a stunning smile.

The weight loss industry has done such a good job of tying our happiness to our weight that we now seem to believe it – as if weight loss were a magical path to happiness.

But it's not. And every time I'd get down to my "ideal weight", I would feel somewhat empty inside and wonder isn't this supposed to make me happy?

When the happiness didn't come, the weight would come back, and I would find myself even more miserable. It wasn't until I learned to be happy, regardless of my weight, that I was able to successfully lose weight.

I believed I needed to punish myself to lose weight

When we think of the words "diet" and "weight loss" the third word that usually comes to mind is "misery." Eating nothing but rabbit food, dry chicken and broccoli, or subsisting on some hardly-edible liquid meal seem to be prerequisites for weight loss. Because everyone else was suffering to lose weight, I needed to suffer too. And if it wasn't painful, it obviously wouldn't work... or so I thought.

I had to believe that my body was flawed, broken, and couldn't be trusted

Because dieting involves sticking to a set plan "come hell or high water" (yes, a trainer said that to me once), I learned not to listen to my body and that my mind knew better. I believed that I had to eat every two hours even though I wasn't hungry, or I had to wait until the next planned meal even when I was ravenous. If my body got me into this mess, I would use my brain instead to get me out.

Beyond believing my body was not to be trusted, I also started to buy into the belief that it was broken and flawed. I Believed I was carb intolerant, gluten intolerant, adrenally challenged, hormonally unbalanced, "toxic"… anything and everything that could be cured by a "miracle supplement" or extreme diet… although the supposed cure never seemed to work.

These beliefs were not only damaging my weight loss progress, but they were also destroying my life. The belief that I couldn't be trusted carried over to my professional life where I started second-guessing my decisions at work. The idea that I had to suffer bled into my personal life, leading to some pretty bad relationships. The notion that I couldn't be happy unless I was thin destroyed every aspect of my happiness.

At some point, I realized that something had to change. These beliefs were more toxic to my life than any food could ever be!

I set my goal of weight-loss-at-any-expense aside and focused on re-establishing some positive beliefs. Here are the beliefs I chose to adopt and incorporated into my life:

I can be happy at this moment, regardless of my weight

The fact is happiness is not a number on the scale, just like it is not the size of a house or the number in a bank account. Despite what our culture has taught us from our youth that "if you work hard now you'll be happy later, " happiness doesn't from achieving some socially accepted idea of success, but from fully embracing and living in the present.

Weight loss and healthy eating is about nourishing myself and not about punishing myself

When we hate our bodies, all we can think is: what can I do to change them? Once I learned to love myself and be happy, regardless of my weight, I started asking a different question: what can I do to nourish my body? By focusing on nourishing myself, instead of punishing myself, I naturally began to want to make better choices, without requiring super-human willpower or someone holding my feet to the fire.

My body is a miracle and I can be trusted

The hardest thing I did was to start trusting my body, and eat because I was truly hungry, and not because some diet told me I could. But after years of withholding what my body was asking for, I wanted a trusting relationship with my body. We don't ever withhold oxygen from our bodies because we think we should go with less. Our bodies are optimally adapted to provide us with what we need: our hearts beat without us having to control it, our lungs breathe without needing to be controlled, why would eating be any different?

Once I adopted these beliefs and began acting on these beliefs, amazing things happened. My body communicated what it needed: Once I asked myself if I was truly hungry or not–a question I hadn't asked since my high school days when I began restricting my eating—I began getting very clear signals. Not only was I more in tune with what my body needed to eat, but also with how much rest, relaxation, and hydration I needed.

I also found myself easily making better food decisions. Because I was no longer punishing myself and was focused on nourishing myself instead, I created a deep desire to eat foods that helped me feel great, met my needs, and also tasted delicious. And what's amazing is that, even though chose to be happy regardless of my weight, I did lose weight, and kept it off, seemingly effortlessly.

If you are struggling to lose weight or maintain your health and fitness results, I urge you to consider the mind set with which are you approaching your weight loss goals. Most of the diet industry promotes a negative mind-set that can't possibly lead to success. Instead, adopt positive beliefs and positive motivations for yourself. You may be surprised how easy it is to make better choices when you're encouraging yourself and loving yourself, as opposed to beating yourself up all the time.

Take snapshots and make sure to track everything

Post your day one photos and continue with this habit by trying to post at least once every week, preferably on Monday. Do this to keep you motivated and encouraged. In the case where you are not too good at taking photos ask a friend or relative to help you out.

The photos you take should look like those shown below

- Side view

- Front view with your face forward

- Back view with your back facing the camera

With the help of this, input how much weight you expect to lose every week, to track your daily calorie intake.

Rest and Recover to Sustain Progress

Resting is one part of the process of transformation that most people seem to take for granted, without realizing that it is imperative to the overall success of the transformation procedure. A lot of individuals think that by pushing their bodies to the extreme day in day out, they are conditioning their body to a higher level of physicality in a much shorter time. This belief though substantiated is dangerous as such practice only tricks your body to learn to adapt to such impetuous habit.

The truth is that rest is crucial for healthy muscle growth, without rest muscle tissue has no time to recover from the strain imposed on it during exercise, which will eventually lead to fatigue. This proves that personal growth and improvement are not only influenced by only Gym workouts but also by your ingrain habits. Regimes like hard lifting and physical exertion are sure to stress the body, and even though there are nutritional supplements that could bolster your resistance to stress, it is usually not enough to make up for all the exercise effectuated pro-inflammatory processes and micro muscle tears.

Try as much as possible to maintain a schedule of 7-9 hours' sleep every night, and don't pass up on the chance to rest on non-working days.

Work Hard As hard work reaps dividends

It is common for individuals to get distracted in the gym, don't let that be your case. When at the gym, do what brought you to the gym. During gym sessions take the advice of your trainers seriously and with the aid ensure that you are working within the range of the prescribed intensity levels.

A workout regime that is treated with indifference will most often than not fail; it is important that you treat your sessions and exercise training with utmost importance. And don't forget to take short breaks in between sessions to allow your body to recover.

Keep Track of weekly Weight

In as much as exercise promises a substantial weight loss percentage, the process itself is not instantaneous, it takes up to 72 hours for your body to catch up and respond to impacts of training and diet modifications and even then the visible effects are often meagre. So if you are expecting a drastic change within a very short period, you are only putting yourself on a pedestal for disappointment.

This is why you should keep track of your weekly weight and not your daily weight, as your daily weight is subject to fluctuations and influence from a host of factors that include but are not limited to bowel movements, water weight, and the time of the day.

Reassure yourself that you can do it

The process of transformation and weight loss is a daunting one that requires you to engage in a slow-burning regime that gets tougher by the day.

It is most likely that you would experience challenges on the way. However, a positive outlook helps you to overcome these challenges and reach your long-term goals.

In the event of your success, you are sure to be a source of inspiration to others, and your healthy habits and living will come off as contagious to your friends and family. So anytime it feels overwhelming just remember these facts and never assume something cannot be done without trying it out yourself.

Transform your body and invariably your life for the better, and memories of the past you shall flicker away, leaving you to a healthy and prosperous future.

CHAPTER – 22

Some of the Workout Tips

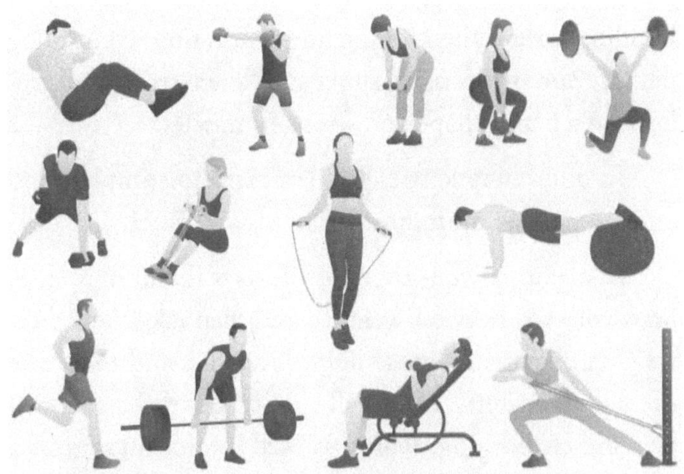

After all the discussion now we need to do some thinking on workout and its process forms in detail.

To transform the body or to build muscle mass, hit one body part a week. If time is premium work alternate, muscles on the same day-like chest and shoulder or back and biceps or shoulders and triceps.

Men who weight train 30 minutes or more daily for a week have a 23 percent lower risk of heart disease than those who don't. Weight training helps increase muscles muscle mass, metabolic rate, and better glucose control reducing the risk of heart dieses.

Free weight offers versatility, but they require good balance and control. Dumbbell and barbell, workouts, call for good, form, more concentrations and in response, these exercises strengthen multiple muscles and stimulate growth.

One of the biggest myths in muscle building is building up and then toning down. It is time-consuming painful and tedious. Shaping and then sizing muscles leads to a better shape and stronger muscles.

To build muscle strength, you need to stimulate and fatigue the maximum number of muscle fibres.

To maximize your training efforts workout in reverse. Start with the heaviest weights, and then take the lighter weights. Eventually those lighter weights, and then take the lighter weights. Eventually, those lighter weights will be more challenging. Warm-up well before you start.

Good form is secret to hitting the target's muscles and stimulates growth. Always keep your eyes straight ahead and your shoulders level. Your body will automatically fall into the proper position and you won't suffer back strain.

Pausing at different points while you are lowering your weight can make you stronger. The pause keeps your muscles under continuous tension longer and increases the load at various points in the range of motion means greater gains in size and strength.

A strong pair of legs can help strengthen your entire body. Squats lunges and step-ups are the best moves for building leg strength. But don't neglect the leg curl and leg extension, machines. This helps buttress your quads and hamstrings which in turn will protect your knees. No gym? Several times a week do a basic leg extension: Lie down with knees bent and together, feet flat on the floor. Extended and straighten one leg, squeezing quads at the top of the move. Alternate legs and repeat for 10 counts.

Instead of popping a pain killer to ease post-workout soreness, take a cold shower. Cold water constricts the blood vessels in the muscles and reduces inflammation and soreness.

An average middle-aged person's problem is not excess weight as much as excess body fat. Simply losing weight is wrong. The key is to change the inactive energy source fat to active tissue muscles. Active tissues burn more calories.

Stretching helps the body rid itself of the chemical build-ups that cause muscle soreness. No one likes to walk like Frankenstein after a workout.

As you grow older your muscles become more resilient. Two days weekly sessions are generally the best options to keep your firm. Try going for more repetitions with low weights.

Never miss a Monday workout. Exercising on the first day of the week sparks a chain reaction in your workout routine that keeps your going through the week.

You get more than a hangover after a night of heavy drinking. 35 percent of your muscle growth gets impaired!

Squats-thrust push-ups get you in great shape because they work your upper body, core, and lower body and improve agility, strength, and endurance all at once.

Working out with a ball, an exercise ball is a great asset. It adds balance and flexibility to your workout. Though used for abdominal workouts, it exercises muscles in the thighs buttocks sides, and back too.

The secret to a flatter, firmer tummy is to combine abdominal exercise with a sensible low-fat diet. For best results mix up your routine with exercise that targets the various muscles that make up your abdominal area.

For well-toned hamstrings take up aerobic activities such as speed walking and spinning/cycling. Combine it with a sensible diet and weight training and you can wish away that flab.

If you suffer from joint anxiety or loose ligaments and tendons around the shoulder and knees, the best way to fix your problem is to strengthen the surrounding muscles.

Jumping rope is a groovy aerobic exercise. It increases heart rate, builds cardiovascular endurance and bone strength, burns a lot of calories, and works out the shoulders, chest, forearms, and lower body. And you can do it even if you have bad knees! Ideally jumping rope should be done after your weight training. This will help increase stamina.

Over time our muscles adapt to any new exercise routine. So mix it up by cross-training with free weights, machines, and resistance band exercise.

Weight lifting improves shortness of breath fatigue anxiety and irritability more than endurance exercise it also helps people feel more in control of their disease.

Boxing and heavy bags work out to maximize fitness level because they work your entire upper body, harden core and abdominal muscles, and give intense cardiovascular results. It's also a nice way to vent out frustration.

CHAPTER – 23

Idea Behind NAGA Fitness

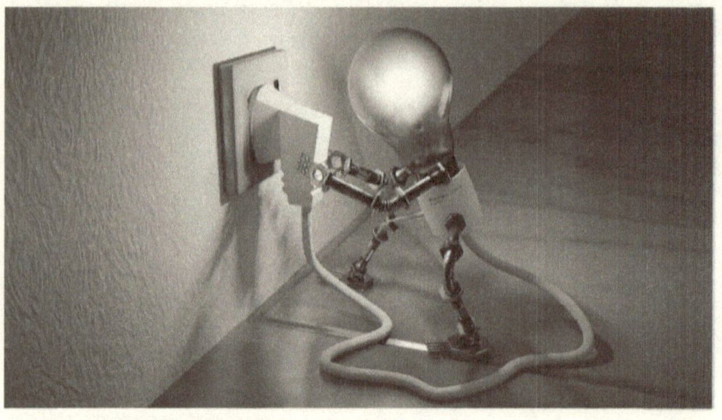

Fitness is altogether a journey towards starting or leaving a fit lifestyle, it includes many things it's a universe. The concept of to start NAGA fitness was resultant of that, first I have transformed me than few more people then socially connected people approached for the same once they start getting results. Some of them motivate me to launch my fitness platform to help people in mass.

Naga Consist of- Nutrition, Attempt, Goal, and Action.

Nutrition:-

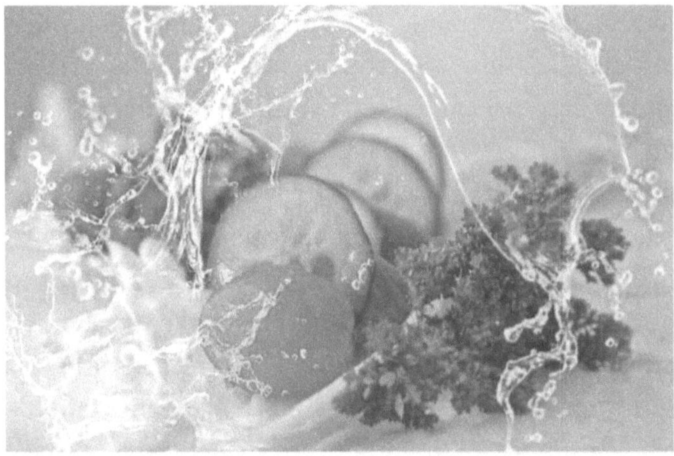

As the name suggests, 'nutrition' includes in itself' nutrients' which can be broadly classified as carbohydrates, proteins, fats, vitamins, minerals, roughage, and water. A balanced amount of these nutrients in the right proportions constitute a healthy diet. The words' balanced' and 'right proportions' mentioned previously are key to life when it comes to consuming nutrients. 'Optimum Nutrition' is defined as eating the right amount of nutrients in a proper schedule to achieve the best performance and longest possible lifetime in good health. The importance of nutrition can be visibly highlighted by the increasing number of nutrient deficiency diseases such as night blindness, scurvy, cretinism, anaemia, and nutrient excess health-threatening conditions like obesity, metabolic syndrome, and other cardiovascular anomalies.

Undernutrition in underdeveloped and developing countries has been marked by malnutrition due to lack of even the basic staple nutrients causing diseases like marasmus and kwashiorkor. Animal nutrition on the molecular level comes from nitrogen, carbon, and hydrogen compounds. Nutrients are the building blocks of the food chain, which interlink to form food webs and influence world food production via biodiversity. Similarly, plant nutrition is referred to as the chemicals that are necessary for plant growth and other physiological processes in plants like metabolism, transport, photosynthesis, etc. Nutrients essential for plants are obtained from the soil, air, sunlight, and as a whole from the earth; thus, the nutrients can be recycled and renewed, making them easily available for sustenance of life.

Fatigue, tiredness, and apathy are common among the working class as well as students. To feel refreshed, motivated as well as reenergized, all we require is the proper nutrition for our systems. Nutrition helps an individual attain optimal health throughout life as well as boost self-esteem.

Eating a balanced diet improves a person's health and well-being and reduces the risks of major causes of death. The other benefits of nutrition include a healthy heart, strength in teeth and bones, maintains good brain health, boosts immunity, bolsters the body to fight against diseases, keeps higher energy levels, and keeps the body weight in check. With such a minimum as maintaining our diet comes the strength of independence or self-dependence. The topic of nutrition has gained its importance by being studied and researched over for years. Nutrition is taught as a subject in various levels of education, and professions such as farmers, scientists, nutritionists, dietitians, health counsellors, and doctors who form the pillar of our society.

As the name suggests, 'nutrition' includes in itself' nutrients' which can be broadly classified as carbohydrates, proteins, fats, vitamins, minerals, roughage, and water. A balanced amount of these nutrients in the right proportions constitute a healthy diet.

The words' balanced' and 'right proportions' mentioned previously are key to life when it comes to consuming nutrients. 'Optimum Nutrition' is defined as eating the right amount of nutrients in a proper schedule to achieve the best performance and longest possible lifetime in good health. The importance of nutrition can be visibly highlighted by the increasing number of nutrient deficiency diseases such as night blindness, scurvy, cretinism, anaemia, and nutrient excess health-threatening conditions like obesity, metabolic syndrome, and other cardiovascular anomalies.

Undernutrition in underdeveloped and developing countries has been marked by malnutrition due to lack of even the basic staple nutrients causing diseases like marasmus and kwashiorkor. Animal nutrition on the molecular level comes from nitrogen, carbon, and hydrogen compounds. Nutrients are the building blocks of the food chain, which interlink to form food webs and influence world food production via biodiversity.

Similarly, plant nutrition is referred to as the chemicals that are necessary for plant growth and other physiological processes in plants like metabolism, transport, photosynthesis, etc. Nutrients essential for plants are obtained from the soil, air, sunlight, and as a whole from the earth; thus, the nutrients can be recycled and renewed, making them easily available for sustenance of life.

Fatigue, tiredness, and apathy are common among the working class as well as students. To feel refreshed, motivated as well as reenergized, all we require is the proper nutrition for our systems. Nutrition helps an individual attain optimal health throughout life as well as boost self-esteem.

Eating a balanced diet improves a person's health and well-being and reduces the risks of major causes of death. The other benefits of nutrition include a healthy heart, strength in teeth and bones, maintains good brain health, boosts immunity, bolsters the body to fight against diseases, keeps higher energy levels, and keeps the body weight in check. With such a minimum as maintaining our diet comes the strength of independence or self-dependence. The topic of nutrition has gained its importance by being studied and researched over for years. Nutrition is taught as a subject in various levels of education, and professions such as farmers, scientists, nutritionists, dietitians, health counsellors, and doctors who form the pillar of our society are all based on nutrition fundamentals.

Progressive research works from various parts of the world on 'nutrition' have helped in aiding health conditions for the living, yet a big section of society is not reached out for proper food supplies. With the current progressive rate of scientific enhancement in the field of nutrition, resulting in increasing food production, we should be able to reach out to those who are dying due to the lack of something as basic as food, which should be available to everyone equally.

Attempt:-

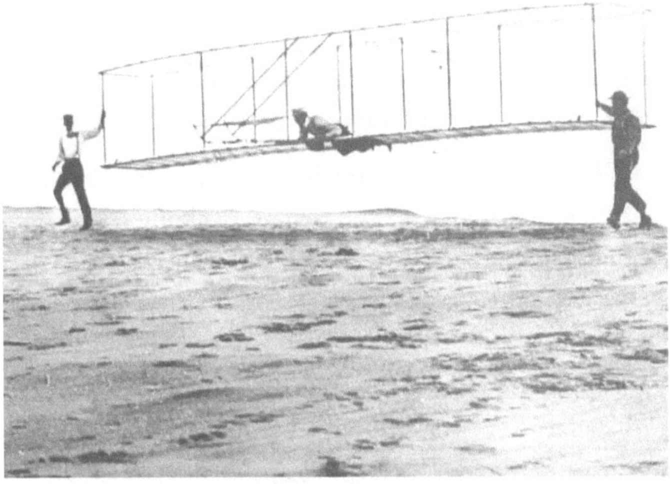

An attempt is something itself saying that you are going to perform some very tough tasks. For that, you need to plan some things and without proper planning, you will not achieve anything.

1. Step Up, Check-Up

If you can't remember the last time you saw your doctor for a complete physical and blood work-up, now is the time. Why? Well, first of all, there's all the disclaimer-sounding stuff concerning any outstanding health issues you might not know about. Your doctor could have specific diet or training recommendations that you're better off hearing about now than later. But that's not the only reason.

Simply knowing where you stand can help your efforts tremendously. In exchange for a few bucks and a little pain, you'll receive health benchmarks on things like cholesterol and triglycerides, blood pressure, fasting glucose, and perhaps bone density for older women. These are concrete, quantifiable areas where you can track progress and see your hard work translate into results.

The scale and the mirror have plenty to say, but they don't tell the whole story. Fitness is about more than looking good; it's about feeling healthy and living well!

2. Take Out The Trash

This applies in all areas of your life: nutritional, mental, and social. Remember, your "before" picture isn't just an image of a body; it's a time capsule portraying all the good, bad, and secret things making up your lifestyle. If you want to put the past behind you, clear out anything in your life that you know will hold you back from success.

Start with the easy stuff. If your cupboards are loaded with cookies, candy, and other junk, clean them out. Having these items around will only tempt you to make poor food decisions. Say goodbye to Oreos and Twinkies.

If you're prone to berating yourself for poor food choices or the way you look, now's the time to make a concerted effort to replace this negative self-talk with more positive statements. Every time a negative statement comes to mind, replace it with two positive affirmations about what you're doing well. This could be something like, 'I chose a healthy chicken salad at lunch today,' or "I drank 10 glasses of water today."

There's no need to focus solely on huge accomplishments like fat loss or muscle gain; progress is progress, and every small victory is significant. Simply focus on what you want to do and shift your entire frame of mind.

Although this might seem callous, similarly take stock of people who could make your transformation more difficult. You need to surround yourself with people who will be supportive, not emotional anchors who drag you down. Especially during the beginning stages of your transformation, you need Adrians, not Paulies. You don't have to break up with anyone; just perform an honest assessment, and then make the most of the people who help you be at your best.

3. Buy The Fundamentals

Let's face it: The world isn't a fit place. If you're relying on the circumstance, gyms, and restaurants to keep you on track, you're going to face an uphill battle. So before you begin, fortify your home base with the essential food and workout arsenal.

Having good choices always at hand in your refrigerator and cupboards will make your life much easier. The specifics will vary depending on the diet play you follow, but these are all solid options to have in your pantry in a pinch.

Pantry Items

- Brown rice

- Quinoa

- Oats

- Sweet potatoes

- Whole-grain cereals

- Nuts

- Natural nut butter

- Sesame seeds

- Olive oil

- Canned tuna

- Salmon

- Spices

Fridge Items

- Fresh fruits

- Greek yogurt

- Egg whites

- Low-fat milk

- Turkey

- Low-sodium soy sauce

- Salsa

- Mustard

- Chicken

- Bottled water

Freezer Items

- Frozen chicken breasts

- Frozen turkey

- Frozen fish

- Frozen vegetables

- Frozen berries

All of these foods can combine to make up your healthful eating plan and provide you with a balanced blend of proteins, carbs, and healthy fats.

You should also have everything you need for simple workouts. Especially if you plan to hit the gym nearly every day, it's a good idea to have some equipment for those rainy days when leaving the house isn't an option. And let's face it: Buying some basic workout items will make your jump into the fitness world more fun. This might sound trivial, but having clothes you like can influence your desire to train.

Training Items

- Properly fitting running shoes

- Comfortable workout wear (bottoms/top/sports bra)

- Music/streaming device

- Water bottle

- Towel

- Heart rate monitor (if desired)

- Jump rope

- Resistance bands

- Dumbbells or kettlebells

Take time to select quality products that will last throughout your transformation.

4. Light Beginner Workouts

Particularly if you haven't exercised in a long time, some light at-home workouts will prime your body and mind for the upcoming challenge. They'll also make you feel more comfortable when you stroll into the gym. Start these workouts as soon as possible, and use them for 1-2 weeks as you get everything ready for your transformation.

Cardio Training

Exercises you should add to your circuit:

- Push-ups

- Decline push-ups

- Assisted pull-ups (or bodyweight if possible)

- Chair dips

- Bodyweight squats

- Walking lunges

- Stationary lunges

- Step-ups

- Glute bridges

- Lying leg lift

- Crunches

- Oblique crunch

- Reverse crunch

Light cardio workouts will help get you accustomed to the exertion you're going to experience over the coming months. Select your favourite method of cardio training—even just some brisk walking will work—and aim to do it 15-30 minutes per day, 3-5 days per week.

Strength Training

It's also a good idea to get started with some basic strength training at home before you begin training at the gym. Bodyweight exercises are an excellent way to learn the essential movement patterns and discover how it feels to train your muscles. Take the time to learn to do them right, and you'll discover they're surprisingly tough!

To start, perform a circuit of four or five different bodyweight movements, aiming for 10 reps per exercise and three rounds of the circuit. Take 30-60 seconds to rest between each circuit. Pick one exercise per body part to build a full-body workout.

Treat this as practice. Switch things up on occasion so that you get better at a variety of movements, but try to improve your form on classics like push-ups, pull-ups (or an appropriate regression, and bodyweight squats. When you're ready to battle heavier weights, you want to have these fundamentals in your corner.

5. Don't Sabotage Yourself

Even when you start going to the gym every day, what you do outside of it will significantly impact your results. If you aren't living well, you won't hit your goals.

Want to know how to live better? First off, start tracking everything in a log or journal. Keep track of your sleep habits, alcohol consumption, and stress and motivation levels. Each of these will play a significant role in your success.

Sleep is critical to muscular repair, maintaining a healthy metabolism, and making sure you feel energized to perform during each training session. If you aren't currently getting at least 8 hours per night, start making that a top priority. You will feel the difference.

No matter if you overindulge on the weekends or just have a couple of drinks in the evening, alcohol is still a toxin. It will negatively affect your ability to burn fat and recover from workout sessions—this much is known. So as much as possible, remove alcohol from the picture, at least during your transformation. Many, many people have discovered after going dry for a few weeks that it was the missing piece of the puzzle for them.

Stress causes trouble for all of us. But for those interested in transforming, high levels of stress can put a damper on your progress. It can have behavioural implications, such as increasing your risk of overeating and skipping workouts, but it's also just bad for your body on several levels. Utilize constructive stress management techniques like journaling, meditating, talking to a friend, or going out for a long drive around the city. Learn what works for you and then put it to use.

Adding a social component to your training is a great way to help you tie it all together and stay accountable for the long haul. Find a buddy, join a class, hire a trainer, join a NAGA Fitness.com group, or make a list of your goals and share it with a loved one. Better yet, do all of the above. Do whatever it takes to fully commit. That is your mantra now: "Whatever it takes."

6. Set Goals

You need goals. We all do. But when you're sore, hungry, and about to start a difficult workout, you'll especially need them—and you'll need them to be relevant to you.

Transformations have both physique and performance dimensions, so it's ok to have goals in both areas. Losing weight, gaining muscle, and looking good in the mirror are examples of the former; squatting 10 more kg, running a km in under 10 km, or finally getting your toes up to that bar are examples of the latter. Having both types of goals will help keep you motivated even if one goal starts to slow in progress.

If your goals are health-related or personal is also important. In fact, for many people, they're more motivational than physique or performance goals. Want to have more energy to play with your kids? Write it down. Want to get those triglycerides to a level where your doctor isn't bugging you anymore? That's a great target.

The more you have to work toward, the greater your chance of success.

7. Begin!

Your gloves are on and you're in the ring. Let the transformation begin! If you're following a particular program, make sure you read up on the details and are familiar with exactly what you're expected to do. Many have gone where you're going, so it's highly likely they've already found answers to the questions you'll be asking.

No matter what comes next, you've made progress simply by deciding to hold yourself to a higher standard.

G- Stands in Naga is goals:-

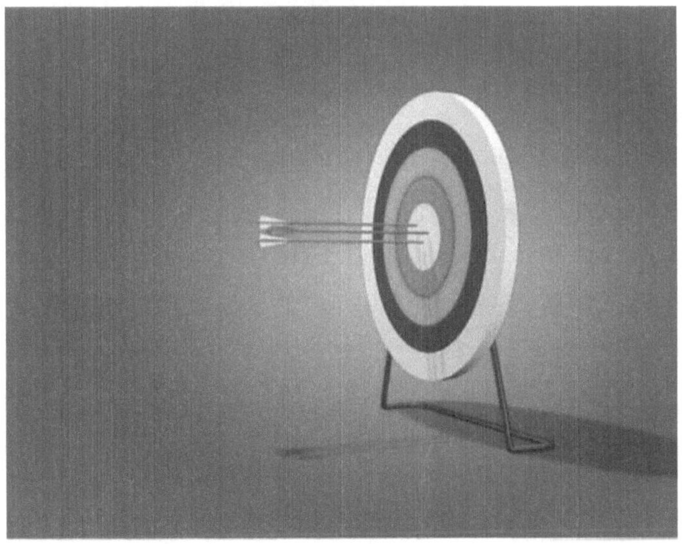

Settings' goal is important for any transformation. Let's understand is details about settings goals in any bodyweight transformation.

Fitness goals are important on several counts. They hold us accountable, expand our definition of possible, and encourage us to push through temporary discomfort for longer-lasting change. But figuring out how to set fitness goals you'll want to attain can be part science. Experts says a good fitness goal can be "your North Star when you have bad days," In other words, a goal, if thoughtful and well structured, can give you the extra incentive to keep going when motivation wanes, or when life otherwise gets in the way.

The problem is that during this time of year, it's easy to get caught up in the rush of New Year's resolutions and set goals that are too lofty, unsustainable, and otherwise unrealistic. We then fail to achieve them and feel worse about ourselves than before we started. This year, to avoid that detrimental downward spiral altogether.

1. Focus on one goal at a time

When it comes to setting a fitness goal, one of the biggest mistakes is that people try to do too much at one time. Perhaps you want to hit the gym every day, cut out added sugar, and get at least eight hours of sleep a night. Trying to tackle that much at once is essentially just setting yourself up for failure. With so many things to achieve, "people get anxious, and if they didn't do one thing, they feel like a failure," This can lead to negative self-talk that lowers your chances of achieving any of the goals.

Instead, pick one thing you want to crush—like, doing a pull-up, or completing your first-ever 5K—and channel your efforts into achieving that before exploring another goal.

2. Make it your own

It can be easy to scroll through the 'gram and feel inspired-yet-envious by images of the super fit. Yet basing your own goals off of what you see others achieving is neither productive nor practical.

When we are bombarded by images of what fitness should look like and how we should do XYZ, it can be hard to identify what's good for you?? Certain things that top athletes can do—run a marathon, do 100 push-ups, master the most challenging yoga poses— "may be great for them, but it's not metric that everyone should be measured by," In other words, your goal should be your goal—something that you are excited about and realistically able to achieve—not someone else's.

3. Make it measurable, specific, and time-bound

Having a measurable goal allows you to track your progress, says experts, and the more specific your goal, the clearer the path to achieving it becomes.

Wanting to "be stronger," for example, is a great place to start, but what does that mean to you? Saying you want to increase the number of push-ups you can do makes the goal measurable, and saying you want to be able to do 20 push-ups in one minute makes it specific. On top of that, the goal should be time-bound, as this helps you focus your efforts, develop a more structured plan for actually achieving the goal, and creates a sense of urgency that can be motivating. Examples of measurable, specific, and time-bound goals include being able to deadlift 10 repetitions with 50 pounds in three months, running a 5K nonstop by the end of the year, and correctly performing a pull-up by the start of summer.

A great way to remember this is through the SMART method, which helps you make sure your goal is specific, measurable, attainable, relevant, and timely. Learn more about setting goals using the SMART method here.

4. Set the bar low—at least, at first

Speaking of attainable: "Your goal should seem relatively easy or within reach of what you are doing," Why? If you think it's easy, you have likely already worked through any mental obstacles that could thwart your progress, on the confidence scale, you should be at a 9 out of 10 when it comes to your belief that you'll achieve your goal. The less confident you are, the less likely you will adhere to the steps needed to make it happen,.

Plus, attainable goals help ensure that you start with some all-important wins. "The more success you have in your fitness journey, the more you will stay with it," having this success early on is especially important as it builds confidence that can snowball into long-term results.

5. Play the long game

We all want instant gratification, but it's important to be realistic with the time frame you develop for achieving your goal, "Lasting changes take a while.

Know that "you are never going to make an overhaul in one week," Instead, pick a goal that can be achieved over the course of several months or even a year. A long-term mentality will help you see your goal as a lifestyle change, rather than a quick fix, and you'll be much more likely to adhere to it.

6. Understand what's driving your goal

Sometimes fitness goals are driven by underlying fears, insecurities, or body image issues—like wanting to run a marathon because you were bullied in middle school gym class, or signing up for a CrossFit class because an ex once commented on your weight—and it's important to address these issues rather than assuming achieving your goal will assuage them.

"Depending on what you are trying to accomplish, it can stir up a lot of emotions," If thinking about your goal brings anxiety and/or triggers past mental struggles, consider talking with a mental health professional.

7. Be flexible in your definition of success

Though it is important to make your goal specific, it's also important to permit yourself to alter it as you progress with your fitness journey. Perhaps a goal that seemed appropriately challenging at first is way too tough to maintain, or vice versa.

"If your definition of success is rigid, it will be hard to maintain that," Set goals you think you can achieve and then modify them as you understand more what you are capable of, there's nothing wrong with moving the goalposts as you get more comfortable with your body's abilities.

8. Develop micro goals on the way to your big goal

Within your larger goal, you should schedule smaller, confidence-building goals that are achievable in a shorter period. For example, say you want to run a nine-minute km. During your training, you should make a smaller goal, like running a half-km in five minutes, to both shows yourself how much you've accomplished and assess where you currently are. "It's all about those little victories," "You want to be able to reward yourself mentally." Having to wait too long to feel like you've accomplished anything can diminish your motivation and pull you off track entirely.

In general, it's good to set micro-goals that can be achieved every two to three weeks, That amount of time can help you determine if you're macro goal is realistic and provide the chance to scale things back if needed.

9. Consider a professional's input

If you're having a hard time evaluating your current fitness level, determining what would be a realistic goal, and/or just feeling overwhelmed about the process, it can be helpful to consult an expert, like a certified personal trainer. A professional can help give you guidance on how realistic your goal is and can help you set markers along the way, so you can check in and confirm you are on the right track over time.

A certified personal trainer will ask clients about various factors influencing their lifestyle, including their prior history with fitness (e.g. Have they trained before? Are they a former athlete? Do they have experience lifting weights?), their nutrition, their work and social history (e.g. Do they have a demanding, high-stress job? Do they go out frequently? etc.). These questions aren't to judge; they're to understand, explains. "Once we understand their lives, we can create a program around that works for them."

On top of that, trainer will conduct several athletic tests—like endurance tests and strength tests—to assess someone's baseline level of fitness. Though you can ask yourself these questions and conduct fitness tests on yourself, if you're new to fitness, it may be helpful to get an expert's input.

10. Be honest about your prior and current habits

Asking yourself the tough questions can help you honestly evaluate what's most appropriate for you. Have you been somebody who in the past has crushed several fitness goals and just wants to take it to the next level? If that's the case, you could likely tackle a more complex goal. Like running a long-distance race at a certain pace.

But if you're new to fitness, which of course is okay, you may want to focus on more simple behaviour modifications, like going to the gym a certain number of days a week.

"If you want to see measurable progression, you have to be realistic with what you are currently doing," If your routine doesn't involve any form of exercise, suddenly getting yourself to the gym five days a week—while certainly possible—may not be the most practical or realistic goal.

On top of that, it's helpful to consider what has stopped you from achieving goals in the past. If you have a chronically hard time getting up in the morning, for example, sign up for evening workout classes rather than aiming for those 6 a.m. sessions. Being honest with yourself will help you identify and eliminate barriers before you get started.

11. Plan for a support system

When thinking about your goal, you should also think about who in your life could encourage, motivate, and hold you accountable for it. Then recruit them whenever you need support. "If people you spend the most time with are supportive of your goals, it will make a huge difference.

Last Letter of Naga stands for Actions:-

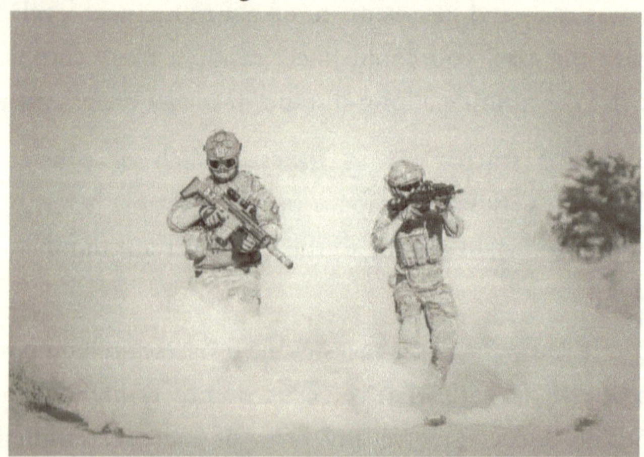

Whatever you have planned to make it work now, the action so let's understand action from NAGA point of view.

Making an action plan

Making an action plan each week can help you plan specific steps for getting more exercise and prepare for things that might get in your way.

Your action plan should be something you want to do, not something you think you should do. Make your plan realistic and action-specific. Make your plan something you can continue to do or build on overtime.

Make your plan something you know you can achieve — be realistic about your current fitness level. Think of exercises you can do now. You can always add on after you achieve your first goal.

Here are some examples of specific and achievable exercise goals:

- I will walk for 30 minutes before work on Monday, Wednesday, and Friday.

- I will work out at the gym for one hour, from 6 p.m. to 7 p.m. on Tuesday and Thursday, and from 10 a.m. to 11 a.m. on Saturday.

- I will add two more laps to my swims this week on Sunday and Wednesday.

Identifying barriers

Once you've figured out your goal, think about what things can get in the way of reaching it. Then figure out ahead of time what things you can do to make it easier for you to reach your goal. Here are some examples:

WHAT MIGHT GET IN MY WAY?

WHAT MIGHT MAKE IT EASIER FOR ME?

I feel rushed in the morning. I'm afraid of missing my bus if I take time for a walk. I'll set my alarm 30 minutes earlier in the morning on Mondays, Wednesdays, and Fridays so I have time for a walk.

I know I can get to the gym on Saturday. But after work, I'm sometimes too tired and just want to go home. I'll tell myself that if I'm too tired when I get to the gym, I'll go home after 30 minutes. I know once I start working out I'll feel great and will be able to go the whole hour.

Creating your plan

Use these tips to make your action plan successful:

- Pick something you want to do.

- Keep your plan realistic. Start with small steps.

- Make your plan action-specific. Know exactly what you're going to do, how much or often, and when.

- Plan ahead for possible barriers and the things you can do to help you succeed.

- Keep track of your progress.

You can use this Action Plan form or create one of your own.

Tracking your progress

At the end of the week, look back on what you've been able to achieve. Congratulate yourself on what went well. Then make a new plan for next week.

You might be able to stretch your goal for next week by doing more of the things that worked. If you fell short of meeting your goal because things got in your way, find solutions that can help you get past your barriers next time. Keeping an activity record may help.

CHAPTER – 24

Why Naga?

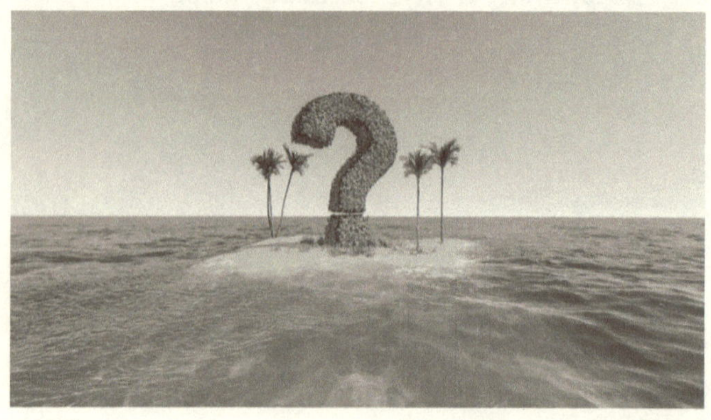

As an online fitness trainer or institution, we think that a good online fitness should have a proper and well-designed fitness plan and program for their client. And with a well-experienced team of a trainer. So we believe and commit below points that we are going to provide these services for sure.

How to Select Online Coach for the workout:-

Along with the other nations, India too has gone digital. Internet as a platform is being used extensively to bridge the gap between the giver and the taker. One such area where the internet has made a remarkable influence is fitness training which has now evolved into Online Fitness Training. With more and more Indians using the power of the internet, online training has already become an applaud able concept. Having a personal trainer around is almost a luxury for a common man who cannot shell out thousands every month on fitness coaching. Hence, a lot of people are ready to give online fitness training a try. Seeking a personal trainer online opens an array of benefits for you including cost-effective training, flexible workout hours, personalization, routines that match your pace, etc. With all this in mind, we have launched our trending online fitness training platform training. NAGA Fitness.com. That aims to assist health enthusiasts in reaching their fitness goals in a simple, systematic, and supportive way.

As fitness trainers, we understand very well how crucial it is to choose the correct mentor. This task becomes all the more difficult when you are going for an online training module. How should you get started with online training? How should one validate online fitness training or trainer? How one should choose an online trainer? These are some of the questions that you must be asked to make the correct choice. Today here, we will assist you in seeking answers to these questions.

Your Fitness Goal:-

You will never be able to find the correct answers to your fitness requirements if you are not sure about your result. You need to understand very clearly what your aim behind finding a personal trainer is. Are you aiming for weight loss or muscle gain? Do you want a lean body or a muscular physique? You need to be sure of what you need from your fitness routine. Once you know this, you can begin your search for a trainer that can assist you in the best possible way. If you are unsure of your goal, you won't have any criteria basis on which you would shortlist a trainer nor would the trainer have any end-point in view while de designing your workout plan. So the first thing to do is setting your fitness goal.

Know the training Types:-

Exercising or gyming are pretty vague terms. There are numerous types of exercises available capable of meeting your fitness requirements. Gyming, aerobics, yoga, Zumba, cross-fit, etc. are different forms of routines that are widely followed. If you have a little knowledge about these then narrow down the type of exercise or training you want to undertake. You can always do some research in trying to understand what would suit you better. Go for the training that will keep you interested. For example, if dancing motivates you, then go for aerobics or Zumba. If you enjoy your sessions, you are more likely to hit your goal.

Once, you know the type of exercise or training you want, you can start looking out for a trainer who specializes in that. If you are not sure about the routine, you want to follow then try opting for a trainer who has expertise in more than one genre.

Search and Research:-

Looking for an online trainer can be quite tricky and at times tiring too. However, it is always better to take sufficient time and precautions in doing this rather than settling down for someone incapable. Whenever, you come across a trainer whom you would want to work out with, first of all, check his/her qualification. Ensure that the trainer holds some sort of certification or degree in health and fitness. If your trainer will also be planning your diet chart, then check whether he is qualified as a nutritionist or not.

Secondly, check his experience. How long has he been fulfilling the role of a trainer? A long tenure shows consistency, dedication, and good results. Check out the client testimonials. If he has his own social media page like Facebook or Twitter, then go through them and see what his followers have to say. Some trainers tend to give false information on a personal website like fake photos and fake reviews. On the IBB training platform, we ask the client for thorough feedback on the trainer after completion of the program which is displayed on the website by us so that only authentic information is available about the trainer. Thus, there is complete transparency which helps you in taking the right decision.

Specialty v/s Goal

Every coach has some specialty like weight loss or gain, bodybuilding, sports physique, aerobics, cross-fit, post-injury workout, post-pregnancy sessions, etc. A trainer might specialize in more than one field. What's important here is to see that his specialty matches your goal. You obviously should not choose a trainer that specializes in bodybuilding and muscle gain when all you want to do is lose weight after delivering a child. So check out with care that the trainer's offerings are meeting your needs before the final selection.

Website Analysis:-

The link between your trainer and you will be his website. It is through the website that he will deliver your workout routines, your diet chart in the form of videos (mostly). Do not go for a website that provides instructions as written matter. You will not be able to perform a routine simply by reading the instructions. Check out sample videos available on the website. See how the language and quality of the video are. Check out how descriptive the content is. See whether you can follow the instructions in the sample video easily.

Another important thing that you need to check is how frequently the content is updated on the website. It is ideal to have a trainer who updates his training material on a weekly or fortnightly (every 15 days) basis.

Payment and Service:

Since this is online training; you will be making online payments as well. See whether the payment gateway is secured or not. Go for the websites that give you some flexibility when it comes to making payments. This reduces the chances of it being a fraud. Refrain from websites that ask you to deposit the fee into a personal account. Companies that rely on NEFT or Bank Deposits for payment of charges usually have higher chances of being a hoax. The website should have a payment gateway that is secured to promote safe transactions.

Also, before making transactions, check out what you will get in return. Ensure that the website explains properly what the services offered are. Sometimes the websites provide material in the form of PDFs and Excel that are meaningless when it comes to fitness training. Get in touch with your chosen trainer and ask him for a detailed explanation of the services that will be offered by him. In addition, read the website's refund policy before making transactions.

Trainers Availability:-

It is important to see that your trainer has some sort of process in place through which he can address your concerns and answer your doubts. The website should have contact information so that you can get timely solutions. Many trainers offer 24/7 chat and phone support. Many trainers use social media like Facebook and Twitter to connect with their clients. So before finalizing on the trainer, visit his/her Facebook page and Twitter handle to check out their activities and the promptness in giving replies. If your trainer is vigilant in making himself available for the clients, then he is a good choice.

Elaborative processes

Keep an eye on the registration process. A good trainer will seek as many details as possible from you right in the beginning so that your workout and diet plans can be made to suit your needs. If the trainer is not keen on knowing about health history and requirements, then it is safe to assume that he is not serious about being an instructor. Similarly, a good trainer will also have different modules for different clients. He will customize the routines to suit his clients' individual needs. If his modules show no personalization, then you might want to look for another coach.

These are a few parameters that can help you in analysing an online coach. You might feel this is a lot of work but try to look at it as a one-time investment. Looking at all the benefits that online personal training has to offer this effort is worth taking.

So We at Naga provide all the above services.

Why NAGA?

As an online fitness trainer or institution, we think that a good online fitness should have a proper and well-designed fitness plan and program for their clients.

How to Select Online Coach for Workout: Seeking a personal trainer online opens an array of benefits for you including cost-effective training, flexible workout hours, personalization, routines that match your pace, etc. With all this in mind, we have launched our trending online fitness training platform, **NAGAFitness.com.**

Your Fitness Goal: Are you aiming for weight loss or muscle gain? Do you want a lean body or muscular physique? You need to be sure of what you need from your fitness routine.

Know the Training Types: There are numerous types of exercises available which are capable of meeting your fitness requirements. Gym exercises, aerobics, yoga, Zumba, cross-fit, etc. are different forms of routines that are widely followed.

Search and Research: Looking for an online trainer can be quite tricky and at times, tiring too. However, it is always better to take sufficient time and precautions in doing this rather than settling down for someone incapable.

Specialty v/s Goal: A trainer might specialize in more than one field. What's important here is to see that his specialty matches your goal.

Website Analysis: The link between your trainer and you will be through your trainer's website/app. Do not go for a website that provides instructions as written matter. You will not be able to perform a routine simply by reading the instructions.

Payment and Service: Since this is an online training, you will be making online payments as well. See whether the payment gateway is secured or not.

Trainers Availability: It is important to see that your trainer has some sort of process in place through which he can address your concerns and answer your doubts.

Elaborate Processes: Keep an eye on the registration process. A good trainer will seek as many details as possible from you right in the beginning so that your workout and diet plans can be made to suit your needs.

www.ingramcontent.com/pod-product-compliance
Lightning Source LLC
Chambersburg PA
CBHW051057250726
48656CB00001B/338